W9-CBK-388

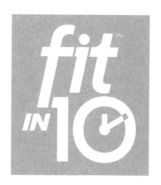

SLIM & STRONG
for Life!

Simple Meals and Easy Exercises for Lasting Weight Loss in Minutes a Day

JENNA BERGEN SOUTHERLAND

Prevention FITNESS DIRECTOR

RODALE.

MONROEVILLE PUBLIC LIBRARY
4000 Gateway Campus Blvd.
Monroeville, PA 15146-3381

LIBRARY

DEC 1 ? 2017

MONROEVILLE, PA

For every woman who has ever
hoped for better and felt overwhelmed
about how to get there.

And for my family, whom
I love to the moon and stars.

© 2017 by Rodale Inc.

All rights reserved. No part of this publication may be reproduced or transmitted in any form
or by any means, electronic or mechanical, including photocopying, recording, or any other
information storage and retrieval system, without the written permission of the publisher.

Rodale books may be purchased for business or promotional use for special sales.
For information, please e-mail: BookMarketing@Rodale.com.

Prevention is a registered trademark of Rodale Inc.

Printed in the United States of America

Rodale Inc. makes every effort to use acid-free ∞, recycled paper ♻.

Recipe photos—Front cover: (top left) Grilled Steak and Avocado Tacos, page 221,
and (bottom right) PB and J Oatmeal Cup, page 176; Back cover: (middle left) Banana Peanut Butter
"Ice Cream" Parfait, page 226, and (bottom left) Portobello Turkey Burger with Bruschetta, page 191

Matthew Rainey/Rodale Images (before and after portraits): pages 9, 17, 25, 37, 45, 129, 145, 155

Grace Huang (portraits): pages iv (photo 1), xii, 8, 30, 36, 46, 128, 154

Mitch Mandel/Rodale Images: all other photos

Food stylist for the recipe photos: Adrienne Anderson

Prop stylist for recipe photos: Karin Olsen

Decorative art: ©Vera Petruk/Getty Images; ©Juan Facundo Mora Soria/Getty Images

Recipes by Rodale Test Kitchen

Book design by Carol Angstadt

Library of Congress-in-Publication Data is on file with the publisher

ISBN 978-1-62336-907-1   direct hardcover

ISBN 978-1-62336-995-8   trade paperback

Distributed to the trade by Macmillan

4   6   8   10   9   7   5   3   direct hardcover

2   4   6   8   10   9   7   5   3   1   trade paperback

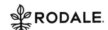

RODALE.

We inspire health, healing, happiness, and love in the world.
Starting with you.

RODALE *wellness*

Live happy. Be healthy. Get inspired.

Sign up today to get exclusive access to our authors, exclusive bonuses,
and the most authoritative, useful, and cutting-edge information on health, wellness,
fitness, and living your life to the fullest.

**Visit us online at RodaleWellness.com
Join us at RodaleWellness.com/Join**

This book is intended as a reference volume only, not as a medical manual.
The information given here is designed to help you make informed decisions about your health.
It is not intended as a substitute for any treatment that may have been prescribed by your doctor.
If you suspect that you have a medical problem, we urge you to seek competent medical help.

The information in this book is meant to supplement, not replace, proper exercise training.
All forms of exercise pose some inherent risks. The editors and publisher advise readers
to take full responsibility for their safety and know their limits. Before practicing
the exercises in this book, be sure that your equipment is well-maintained, and do not
take risks beyond your level of experience, aptitude, training, and fitness.
The exercise and dietary programs in this book are not intended as a substitute for any
exercise routine or dietary regimen that may have been prescribed by your doctor.
As with all exercise and dietary programs, you should get your doctor's approval before beginning.

Mention of specific companies, organizations, or authorities in this book does not
imply endorsement by the author or publisher, nor does mention of specific companies,
organizations, or authorities imply that they endorse this book, its author, or the publisher.

Internet addresses and telephone numbers given in this book were accurate at the time it went to press.

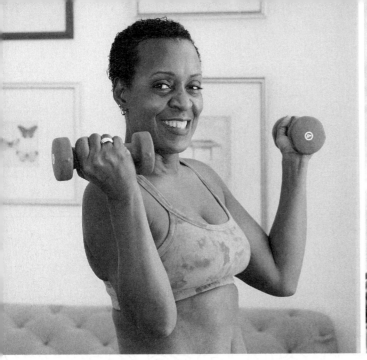
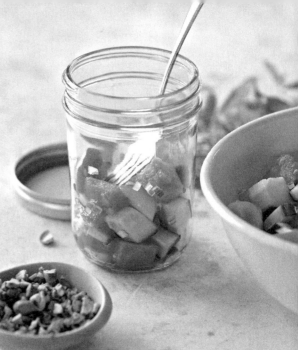

Contents

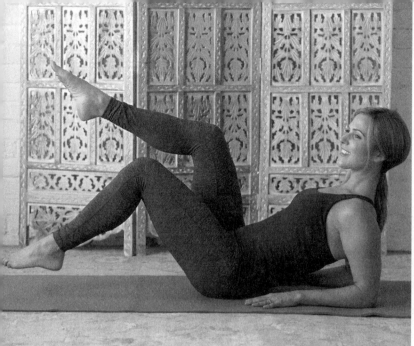
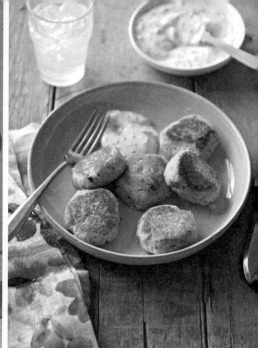

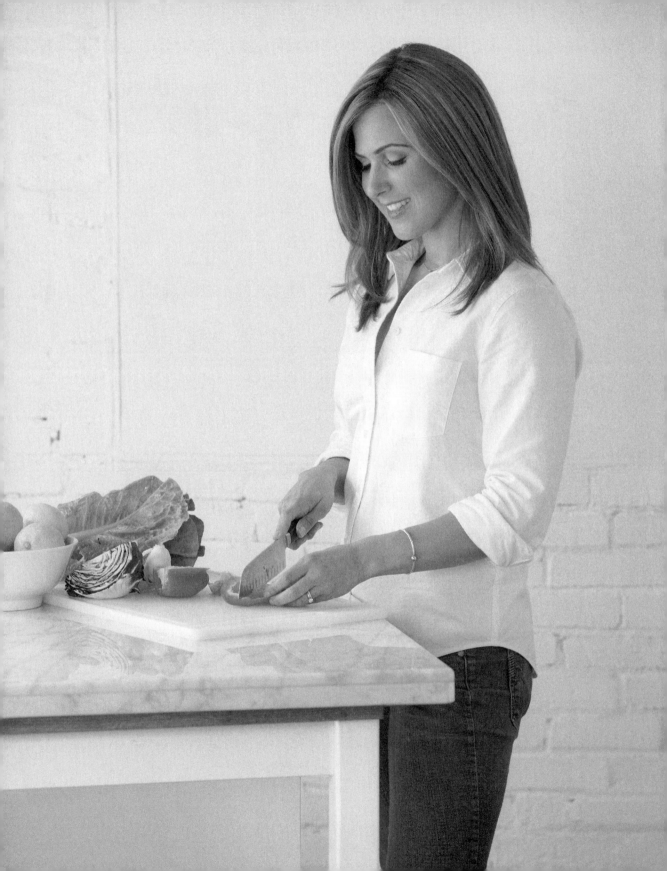

Life Is Complicated.
Fit in 10 Is Simple.

"I'm healthier, I have so much more energy, and for the first time in a very long time, I'm finally showing up for my life again," says the woman standing in front of me. The 59-year-old New Yorker barely resembles the person that I met just 60 days earlier. She's lighter now, and not just physically.

When I first met Lori Lowell, she was exhausted. Desperate to feel better, she had applied to be part of the *Fit in 10: Slim & Strong—for Life!* test panel. It wasn't just the long hours she put in at work. Her job as an office manager of a medical office was taxing, and the 12-hour days didn't leave her much time for herself, but for the most part, she enjoyed it.

No, it wasn't work. It was everything else. First, she was physically run down. She hadn't gotten a decent night's sleep in months. Her back ached so badly that every time she turned over in bed, the pain woke her. She'd always struggled with her weight, but she'd never been this heavy before. The last time she got on a scale, the number she saw—190 pounds— shocked her. It was too much for her 5-foot-6 frame. Plus, ever since she turned 50 and the hormonal storm hit, she wasn't just carrying it in her hips and thighs. Now, it had settled around her belly, making it much harder for her to do the gardening she enjoyed and to find clothes that fit.

On top of feeling physically awful, Lori was mentally drained. Her younger sister, Donna, was battling brain cancer, her father-in-law was in the early stages of Alzheimer's, and she and her husband, Ken, were still trying to get two of their three kids through college. It was just too much.

"I'm so sick of feeling overwhelmed and out of shape," she'd told me. "I need to make a change that's actually sustainable."

10-Minute Transformations

My heart ached for Lori during that initial conversation; I understood the very real hurdles she was up against. But I also felt hopeful for her, because I knew there was a simple solution that would help her turn around her health and get back in shape in just minutes a day.

Over the last 3 years, Fit in 10 has empowered thousands of busy women to lose the stubborn weight that was slowly eroding their health and stealing their joy. Without dieting. Without punishing their bodies with ridiculously tough workouts.

I never grow tired of seeing someone's face light up when she learns that she doesn't have to suffer through miserable diets or torturous exercise to feel good in and at peace with her body. That moment when she realizes she can enjoy amazing food while living the life she wants in the healthy body she needs. When the cloud lifts and she gives me a hug, her eyes bright, and she says, "Thank you. For everything." I squeeze her back, feeling humbled and lucky to have met another Fit in 10 soul sister who inspires me to continue to prioritize my own health and wellness.

If you're reading this book, you probably know how exhausting it is to feel uncomfortable in your body or to think constantly about your weight and stress over what, exactly, you should be eating. You also know how crummy it

is to feel guilty about missing yet another workout. The truth is, most of us already have a general understanding of what we should be doing to stay healthy and strong—eat better, move more—but we get lost in the details and overwhelmed by "How in the world am I ever going to find the energy or time to do it all?"

I know, because I've been there, too.

A Desire for Something Easier

The idea for Fit in 10 started brewing when I began to realize that my time-crunched life was only going to get busier. Here I was, the fitness director of *Prevention*, blessed with an abundance of wonderful opportunities to do a job I believed in and loved, and yet I was struggling to find a way to fit in all of the good stuff I knew I was supposed to be doing. I spent most of my days parked in front of a computer and most nights, after walking in the door after 7 p.m., scrambling to get a clean meal on the table before falling into bed and doing it all over again the next day.

It was also getting harder and harder to squeeze in my daily runs and twice-a-week yoga classes, let alone get to the strength-training workouts I knew my body and metabolism needed to stay strong and youthful. Every expert I spoke to and countless new studies backed the importance of lifting weights, and I wrote and edited numerous stories for *Prevention* on why every woman needed to be doing more of it. Still, while I made it to the occasional boot-camp class, I was largely part of the 80 percent of American women who weren't strength training regularly.[1]

When I hit my midthirties and my body started to lose tone and feel achier, I promised myself over and over that this would be the week when I was finally going to start making strength training a priority. Then, reality would set in and I'd be crushed by a wave of deadlines, e-mails, and millions of other little must-dos, and my goal to get stronger and leaner would be washed away. I remember thinking to myself, "I don't even have kids yet. This is only going to get harder!"

As someone who struggled with weight in the past, I wasn't about to let my health and fitness slide backward (you can read more about my "aha moment" on page 22). I had to find a doable solution, one that I could share with every woman who was in a similar struggle. So, I started to wonder, "What's the littlest amount of strength training someone could do each day and see a major difference in her strength and body?" After diving into the research and chatting with some of the top experts in the field, I eventually settled on 10 minutes—the time you could find, say, right before you hop into the shower or while dinner cooks in the oven. Research conveys that 10 minutes of simple movement can make a huge difference in everything from your mood to your metabolism (see page 4 for more). But I chose 10 minutes mostly because I believed it was truly doable. Because if it wasn't simple, there was no way I was going to fit it into my busy life.

When I brought the concept of Fit in 10 to my team at *Prevention,* they loved the idea of such a simple plan, and the wheels were set in motion. After creating the workouts with trainer Larysa DiDio, we tested my fitness hypothesis with real women in the real world. We were shocked by how quickly 10 minutes of metabolism-revving strength training could transform one's body and health when paired with simple, clean eating. We saw it work with women of all ages and fitness levels, whether it was someone like Lori, who needed to ease back into exercise, or someone like me, who needed to add in regular strength training to break through a plateau.

Over the last few years, we've created two successful fitness DVDs—*Fit in 10: Total-Body Transformation* and *Fit in 10: 30-Day Belly Fix*—that have helped women get fit right at home, in just 10 minutes a day. While the workouts were tremendously effective, I kept hearing one very important question from our Fit in 10 community: *When are you going to make clean eating as simple as the 10-minute workouts?*

Making Good Food Simple

The result is the book you are now holding in your hands. *Fit in 10: Slim & Strong—for Life!*

is the first Fit in 10 program that combines new 10-minute toning routines with a cookbook's worth of 10-minute clean meals that will make weight loss easy and enjoyable. This isn't diet food. This is *real* food. These are clean, yummy, homemade recipes that you—and your family—will love. Every meal is as simple to make as it is delicious to eat. You'll find protein-packed breakfasts for your busy mornings, perfectly portable lean lunches, and amazingly simple and satisfying dinners that are a snap to put together after a long day. And of course, since I believe that life's better with dessert, we've included healthy treats that will satisfy your sweet tooth.

You'll also learn the basics of clean eating so that you're empowered to make smarter choices at the store, when you're eating out, when you're standing in your neighborhood bodega, or if you're wandering the airport wondering what the heck you should grab on the go. These are the simple techniques that have given me the freedom to stay at a healthy weight without counting calories or restricting food groups, and I'm so excited to share them with you. They're also the same guidelines that our Fit in 10 test panelists used to transform their life, health, and bodies.

Strong for Life

At this point in our lives, it's not about looking like a supermodel—it's about feeling like a superwoman. There's so much more to us than the size of our thighs, but we do need to be strong, healthy, and confident so we can live our lives with energy and passion. The 10-minute sculpting routines in this book will help you do that, without ever having to leave your home. Each of the 12 routines will show you how to strengthen and tone every "zone" safely and effectively, in a way that works for *your* body. I know because we tested them with women of all ages and fitness levels.

Real Women. Real Life. Amazing Results.

Once we created the *Fit in 10: Slim & Strong—for Life!* plan, we asked 15 women from the New York City area to see how well it worked for them in the real world of crazy schedules, achy bodies, and families full of picky eaters. They ranged in ages from 33 to 60, and each had her own reasons for needing a way to simplify her health and fitness strategy. Some were busy moms in their thirties and forties who couldn't devote larges chunks of time to exercise, and others were women in their fifties and sixties who wanted to go into the second half of life feeling stronger and healthier than they did 10 or 20 years ago.

After 60 days on the plan, our test panelists were thrilled with their results. (You'll find many of their inspiring stories spread throughout the pages of this book.) Overall, they lost an average of 11 pounds and 23 inches, with some women dropping up to 14, 15, or even 18 pounds in only 8 weeks. They also saw their bodies become tighter and leaner, especially in those hard-to-tone areas like the belly, thighs, and upper arms. Many women found the Fit in 10 lifestyle so enjoyable and doable that they plan to keep following it. (Anne Marie Russo was down 26 pounds at press time. See her story on page 129.) While the weight loss numbers were impressive, the transformation they experienced went far deeper. Women who had previously felt weak and beaten down (emotionally and physically) suddenly were doing things they hadn't done in years.

They were running up the stairs without feeling breathless, squatting down to play with their kids or grandkids, jogging instead of walking around the block, and easily lifting heavy suitcases overhead. They were thinking more clearly, their energy was better than it had been in months, and many of their nagging aches and pains had disappeared. What's more, for the first time in years, they felt confident and happy to be in their bodies. They were enjoying getting dressed in the morning. There was no more hiding under blousy tops or squeezing themselves into pants that were uncomfortably tight.

And remember Lori? Now she's down 13 pounds, sleeps through the night, and feels happier than she has in years. "For the longest time, taking better care of myself and losing weight was always on my mind," she says. "It was like the crack in the ceiling that needed to be fixed, or that dent in the car that needed to be repaired. It was always there, and it was wearing me down. The idea of getting back in shape felt overwhelming, but now I know that it doesn't have to be. There are little things you can do that can make a huge difference."

Now It's Your Turn

Anyone who credits Fit in 10 for their transformation was already amazing. This book isn't here to change you or to try and force you or your body into some ridiculous "ideal." It's here to empower you with smart, simple tools that make it much, much easier for you to give your body what it needs in the time you have. So if you're sick of worrying about your weight, feel confused about what to eat, or want to be strong and lean for the rest of your life, this book will help you do it in minutes a day.

Sometimes I still can't believe that such a small idea has helped so many. I'm so excited for you to experience what happens when you stop thinking "I don't have enough time" and start believing "I can move mountains in the time that I have."

Now, let's start the journey together.

Jenna Bergen Southerland
Fitness Director, *Prevention*

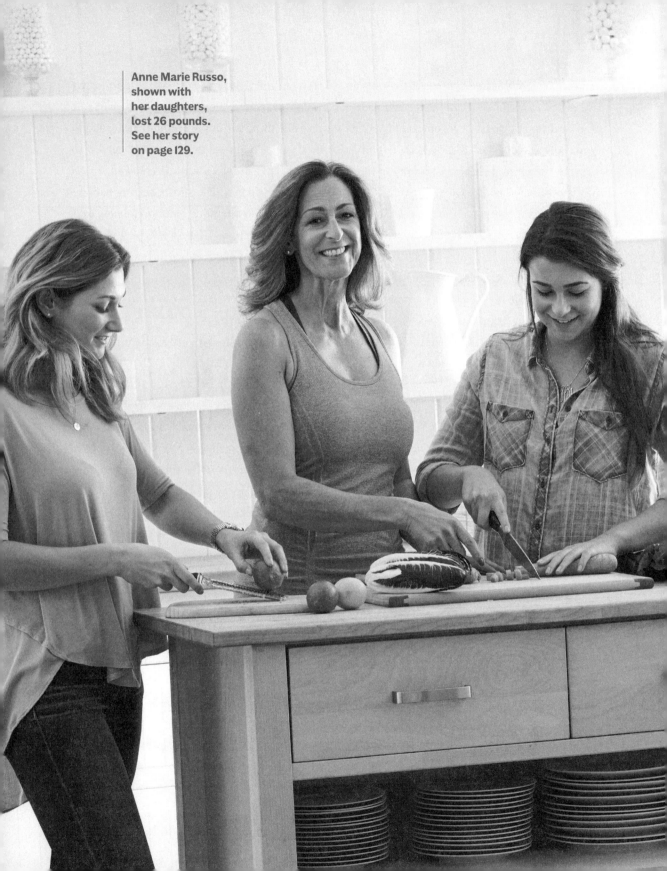

Anne Marie Russo, shown with her daughters, lost 26 pounds. See her story on page 129.

1

The Fit in 10 Lifestyle

If you're thinking, "Really? Just 10 minutes?" you're not the first person to question whether the amount of time it takes to send a few e-mails or to toss in a load or two of laundry can really transform your body and life. Almost everyone who's ever experienced the benefits of Fit in 10 was a little skeptical at first. Even I had doubts whether or not such a tiny chunk of time could actually make a difference before I saw it work first for myself, and then again for hundreds of others.

After all, we've been taught that in order to get what we want, we have to work hard. We have to suffer through awful diets and long, grueling workouts. We have to go crazy counting calories, points, or carbs and put off the things we want to experience in life until we have "more time."

Well, I'm happy to tell you that all of that is *completely untrue.* Once I adopted the Fit in 10 lifestyle, I realized that I didn't have to go through hell to feel good in my body or put off living the life I wanted until things slowed down—and neither do you. I've learned that there is amazing power in focused energy, and while 10 minutes is mini, it's also mighty. Especially when you fill those 600 powerful little seconds with effective strategies that are backed by science.

Need a little more convincing? Here are just a few of the ways that adopting the Fit in 10 mentality will enhance your life, end your weight loss struggles, and make getting and staying in shape easy and enjoyable.

It's Ridiculously Simple

Starting your journey to health as simply as possible makes good sense. After all, you wouldn't jump into trigonometry without having first built a foundation of basic math, would you? The same should apply to how you eat and exercise.

That's why the only thing that's hard about the Fit in 10 program is finding an excuse *not* to do it. It takes the two most challenging parts about getting strong and lean for life—healthy eating and metabolism-revving toning—and makes them so doable and easy to implement that it's kind of a no-brainer. While it's easy for me to shrug off a 60-minute session at the gym, it's really difficult to reason myself out of walking five steps from my computer to the living room and quickly doing 10 minutes of sculpting work. And when a delicious, healthy meal is ready faster than the takeout delivery guy can get to my front door, why cave to processed junk that's only going to make me feel blah the next day? As so many of our test panelists have told me, "You can't argue yourself out of 10 minutes—it's 10 minutes!"

"As a working mom, my life is busy and often complicated," agrees 46-year-old panelist Ali McDowell. "Approaching my health and fitness in 10-minute portions simplified everything and made it much easier to stay consistent and achieve success."

It Reminds You to Make Time for You

Ever been so busy that you glance at the clock only to realize it's 2 p.m. and you haven't even thought about lunch? Or that you've been so caught up in running to meetings, answering e-mails, and putting out fires that you've gone for the last 6 hours without so much as a sip of water? So often we spend our days thinking and taking care of just about everything but ourselves. We're so good at juggling all of it—work, kids, parents, pets, household chores, and everything in between—that we tend to forget about our physical, emotional, and mental needs. Over time, as the stress of the juggle increases, our health and happiness erode like a beach on a rising sea. The result: Our well-being suffers and our overall quality of life plummets.

One of the advantages of the Fit in 10 plan is that it reminds you to put your needs and wants back at the top of your to-do list, 10 minutes at a time. "Now, for the first time in years, the first thing I think about when I wake up is myself," says panelist Anne Marie Russo, 53. "I have to ask myself, 'What am I eating?' 'When can I fit in my 10-minute workout?' It's refreshing to focus on myself and think a little less about everyone else for a change. After all, if I don't do it now, I might not be around to take care of others later."

Many of our panelists also decided to reclaim "me time" in 10-minute chunks. When McDowell told herself she would take just 10 minutes to read—something she loves to do and hasn't done consistently since the whirlwind of motherhood took hold—she was amazed what an impact it had on her mood and stress levels. "The first time I committed to it, I curled up in bed with a book I'd been dying to read and encouraged my daughter to join me with a book of her own," she says. "When the 10 minutes were up, I felt so much more relaxed and was actually able to pay more attention to my daughter. It made me realize that while 10 minutes isn't a lot, it's powerful."

Experts agree: "Many of us are busy, multitasking, and under varying levels of stress. Taking even a small, 10-minute break from the craziness can help us recharge and reduce stress and tension," says Sonja Lyubomirsky, PhD, a professor of psychology at the University of California, Riverside, and author of *The How of Happiness: A New Approach to Getting the Life You Want.* "Research shows that when people are experiencing positive emotions—like joy, curiosity, affection, and tranquility—they are more productive, more connected to others, and have stronger immune function." Then, after the mini refresh, says Dr. Lyubomirsky, we can return to the daily grind relaxed and more prepared to tackle our challenges and embrace life.

It Turns Healthy into a Habit

Our lives are built on routine, whether it's your 6 a.m. wake-up call or the corner coffee shop by the office that you visit almost every afternoon. Sometimes these norms are good for us (like brushing our teeth) and sometimes they're not so good for us (like that 3 p.m. chocolate fix).

While there are nearly countless 21-day programs and apps on the market that promise to help you break bad habits and replace them with better ones in just 3 weeks, research shows that it actually takes a little more than 2 months for most people to adopt new healthy eating and exercise behaviors. Even more interesting: The simpler the task, the faster it tends to become automatic.[1]

That's why the Fit in 10 routines and meal plan are so effective: The time commitment is doable, so you're able to complete the behaviors over and over again until they become natural over the course of 60 days. Then, before you know it, you suddenly have created healthy habits that are your new normal. "That's exactly what happens once you start doing your 10 minutes," confirms 59-year-old test panelist Lori Lowell. "Before I knew it, the routines and recipes had become part of my day. If I didn't have a chance to do my 10-minute workout before I left for work, by the afternoon my body would be restless and I'd start fidgeting at my desk. My

(continued on page 6)

THE SCIENCE OF 10

Research confirms that mini bursts of activity can yield impressive results. Here's what 10 minutes can do for your mind and body.

Speed Up Your Metabolism

Just 10 minutes of exercise fans the flames of your body's fat-burning furnace for at least an hour afterward, according to a study published in the medical journal *Science Translational Medicine*.[2] Researchers at Massachusetts General Hospital took baseline blood samples from healthy women and men and then retook the samples directly following a 10-minute treadmill workout and again 60 minutes after completing the routine. They found that short bursts of activity triggered an increase in more than 20 different metabolites, many of which increased the body's fat- and calorie-burning potential and ability to control blood sugar. What's more, the majority of those metabolites were still elevated an hour after participants had hopped off the treadmill. The researchers also discovered that people who were at a healthy weight saw an even bigger boost—which means that the fitter you get, the bigger payoff you'll receive.

Slim Your Waist

You don't have to spend hours at the gym to score a flatter tummy. In fact, just a few minutes of moderate activity a day can reduce belly fat, according to research published in the *European Journal of Applied Physiology*.[3] At the start of the study, the researchers measured the weight, height, and waist circumference of 42 sedentary Japanese women of ages between 40 and 60 years. They also performed a CT scan of the study participants' abdomens to determine how much subcutaneous fat (the unflattering kind that lies underneath your skin) and visceral fat (the dangerous type that builds up around organs) they were carrying around their bellies. Then, using pedometers, the researchers monitored the women's daily activity levels for 10 days. It turned out that the women who engaged in more frequent sessions of moderate physical activity lasting between 1 and 5 minutes had less visceral fat and smaller waists than women who moved less. Until then, the researchers had hypothesized that in order for exercise to impact belly fat, you had to exercise for more than 10 minutes at a time. Now we know that every little bit counts.

Improve Your Health

Even just three 10-minute workouts a week can pay off big-time for your health, according to a

2014 study published in the online journal *PLOS ONE*.[4] Researchers at McMaster University in Hamilton, Ontario, recruited 14 obese or over-weight men and women who were otherwise healthy to participate in the study. Over the course of 6 weeks, the study participants per-formed eighteen 10-minute workouts on a sta-tionary bike that included just 1 minute of intense interval work. By the end of the study, the participants had increased their VO_2 peak by an average of 12 percent. They also lowered their blood pressure and improved their insulin sensi-tivity. That's all with just three 10-minute work-outs a week—imagine what would happen if you squeezed in 10 minutes each day. Additionally, when sedentary, postmenopausal women added just 10 minutes of light walking a day for 6 months, they significantly increased their overall fitness, according to a study published in the *Journal of the American Medical Association*.[5]

Boost Your Mood

You've heard of a runner's high, but research shows that even 10 minutes of gentle exercise can significantly lift your spirits. Researchers at the Cleveland Clinic had 28 patients with chronic pain rate their perceived level of pain, depres-sion, and anxiety on a scale of 0 to 10 before and after an easy 10-minute walk on the treadmill. Immediately following the walk, the study par-ticipants reported feeling happier and less anx-ious than they had prior to the short burst of exercise. While the perceived levels of pain

remained unchanged immediately following the workout, after 3 weeks of regular exercise the patients' pain levels had dropped by 62 percent.[6]

Additionally, another study, published in the *Baltic Journal of Health & Physical Activity*, found that the mental and emotional benefits of exercise may be felt with even less of a work-out. In fact, just 3 minutes of gentle, standing calisthenics boosted energy and feelings of well-being in college students compared to those who sat quietly for the same amount of time.[7]

Fight Pain

Your desk job may not be physically demanding, but sitting in front of a screen for hours a day can lead to tension headaches caused by a stiff neck and achy shoulders. Thankfully, research shows that lifting weights for just a few minutes a day most days of the week can do wonders for mini-mizing that pain in your head, according to a study published in the *Scandinavian Journal of Work, Environment & Health*.[8] A total of 198 office workers with frequent neck or shoulder pain were randomly assigned to one of two interven-tion groups (resistance training for 2 or 12 minutes a day, 5 times a week) or the control group, which only received weekly health information. At the end of 10 weeks, the group that did 2 minutes of total-body toning had reduced their headache frequency by 43 percent. Those who did 12 min-utes a day fared slightly better, slashing their headache frequency by 56 percent. How's that for a little going a long way?

muscles couldn't wait for me to get home so I could squeeze in a workout."

It Helps You Build Momentum

Every time you make a goal and nail it, you feel awesome, right? Well, with the Fit in 10 program, your goals are so easy to achieve that you get that mini confidence boost multiple times each day. And let me tell you, treating yourself to a 10-minute breakfast before you even leave the house or squeezing in a 10-minute workout in your office while you wait for an e-mail to come through makes you feel pretty terrific. That extra glow doesn't just brighten your mood: A little extra emotional boost can help you stick with healthy habits long-term, according to a study published in the journal *BMC Women's Health*.[9] When researchers interviewed 53 women over the age of 40 about the barriers and facilitators to regular exercise, they discovered something surprising. Weight loss and toning weren't the top reasons that drove the women to get to the gym or squeeze in a walk. Instead, it was the feeling of achievement that they felt every time they followed through on their good intentions to exercise. And when Taiwanese researchers interviewed 12 women who had stuck to an exercise program for 6 months about what kept them going, the women said it was the "continuous power" they built in their mind and body each time

they did a workout or overcame a potential hurdle to exercise (like getting through the initial discomfort) that inspired them to get back to it the next day.[10]

So, basically, every time you do a Fit in 10 routine or eat a Fit in 10 meal, you're more likely to do it again the next day, *and* you get to feel like superwoman. How cool is that?

Not only does your willingness to stick with healthier habits improve as your self-confidence grows, but your mojo to get up and go increases, too.

"As your energy increases and you start to see results, you instinctively build on that momentum," says Wayne Westcott, PhD, a *Prevention* advisory board member and director of fitness research at Quincy College in Massachusetts. "So get out in your garden or walk your dog a little longer—and that extra movement adds up fast."

It Makes Big Goals Doable

It's easy to feel excited at the start of a weight loss program. Your motivation is at an all-time high, you feel unstoppable, and you're envisioning a total transformation—and why not? Then, what happens? You go into crazy mode and set ridiculously hard-to-keep goals, like waking up for a 5 a.m. boot-camp class, white-knuckling yourself off carbs, or finally getting your money's worth out of that juicer

(continued on page 10)

10-MINUTE LIFE CHANGER
Make Your Love List

The Fit in 10 program will help you restore your strength and vitality just 10 minutes at a time. That, however, is just the beginning to a fulfilling life. The second step in creating the life you want is discovering—or perhaps remembering—what brings you happiness and then doing those things! I've found that when my life is a healthier balance between work and pleasure, I have more energy to take better care of myself and I'm less likely to look to food as my main source of enjoyment. So take a few moments now to jot down at least 10 healthy activities or experiences that light you up or bring you true delight. These are what we'll call your First Loves.

Once you have your First Loves down, go a little deeper by asking yourself what it is, exactly, about each of these activities that makes it so enjoyable. For instance, if you wrote down "camping with my family," perhaps the underlying meaning is that you also really enjoy being in nature. So while you should definitely get that camping trip scheduled pronto, that's not something you can probably do every single day (although, if you have a big backyard . . .). So go ahead and mark down "being in nature" as a Second Love. Next, write down the action you will take to start getting those first and second loves into your life. Start seeking out ways to get outside more often—even if that's just walking outside for 10 minutes before lunch or after dinner. Second Loves aren't First Loves, but they're close enough that they will still bring you a shot of joy on a regular basis.

Once you have your list of First and Second Loves, post it where you'll see it often (the fridge, your bathroom mirror, near your desk). Aim to fill yourself up with a Second Love at least once a day (even 10 minutes of "me time" can be powerful; see page 2) and don't put off the First Loves longer than you absolutely have to. Life is short—make it amazing.

EXAMPLE: MY LOVE LIST

FIRST LOVE	SECOND LOVE	ACTION
Vacationing in Paris	Hearing and speaking French	Listening to the free podcast Coffee Break French

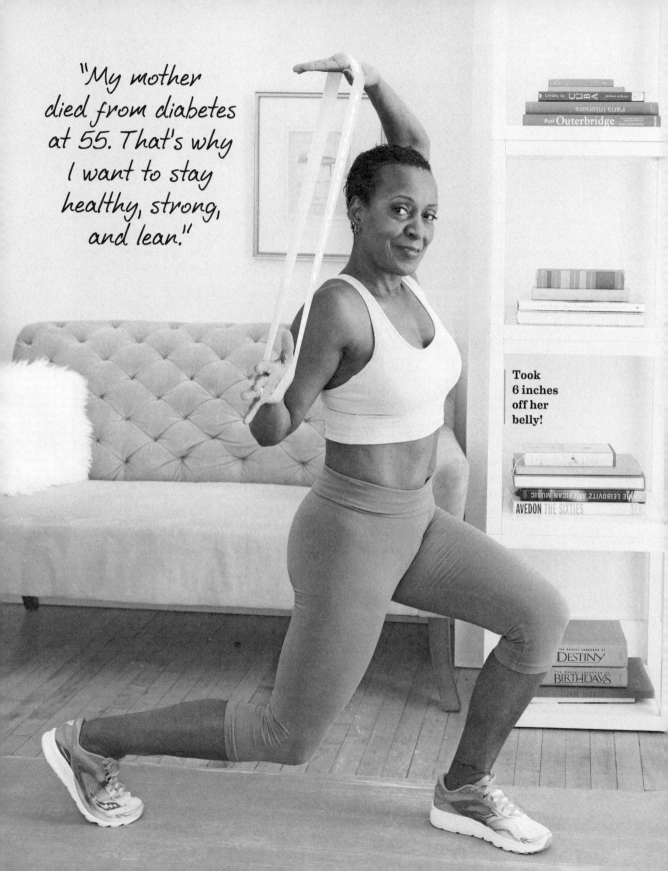

"My mother died from diabetes at 55. That's why I want to stay healthy, strong, and lean."

Took 6 inches off her belly!

Merlyn Joseph

After losing 10 pounds with *Prevention*'s first Fit in 10 DVD program, *Fit in 10: Total-Body Transformation,* Merlyn Joseph understood the power that 10 minutes of daily strength training had on her mood and body. "It makes me feel incredible, like I'm 20 years old again," says the busy New York-based personal chef. So when Merlyn heard about *Prevention*'s new program, *Fit in 10: Slim & Strong–for Life!,* she was eager to try it. "I'd recently taken on a new client, so I was busier than ever, and I'd started slacking on my workouts and diet," she says. "I wanted to lose the few pounds that had crept back on and get back to that place where I have amazing energy. I have eight grandchildren, and I want to be able to run around with them and have fun."

Another goal: Merlyn also wanted to learn how to eat for energy and health, and she was thankful that the Fit in 10 program gave her a simple program she could easily follow. Within days of incorporating the meals and workouts into her schedule, Merlyn knew this was a plan she'd stick with long term. "Not only did I love the food, but the plan taught me how to eat so that I felt energized throughout the day and I was never hungry," says Merlyn. Once she learned how to fuel her body for optimal health, Merlyn realized she hadn't been getting enough lean protein to keep her muscles strong. "I'm a vegetarian, so sometimes it can be challenging to get all of the nutrients my body needs. But the Fit in 10 meal plan showed me how to get enough protein while still staying meatless."

Merlyn also liked that the plan encouraged her to keep track of her meals and workouts.

AGE: **53**

POUNDS LOST: **12**

INCHES LOST: **12**

"Journaling really kept me accountable," she says. "I enjoyed tracking my progress and seeing how far I'd come. It really helped me drop weight quickly. Even when I went on an 18-day trip to Portugal, I didn't gain an ounce of fat."

The new Fit in 10 routines helped Merlyn quickly regain her strength. "I loved that this program incorporated the bands. They toned everything so quickly and gave me amazing endurance," she says. "Now I tell my friends, 'If there's an emergency, baby, you're not catching Merlyn! She's gonna run!'"

By the end of 8 weeks, Merlyn had dropped 7 pounds and was back to her Fit in 10 self. Now, she's down 12 pounds and feeling amazing. "This year I turned 53, and I feel better than I did in my twenties!" she says. "My arms and abs are firmer. When I look in the mirror now I just think, *wow!*"

Of course, Merlyn is quick to remember that it's not just about vanity. "My mother died from diabetes when she was only 55, and before that, she lost a leg from the complications," says

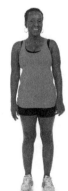

Merlyn. "I don't want my kids to go through what I did with my mom. That's why I want to stay healthy, strong, and lean."

Why Merlyn Loves Fit in 10

THE FOOD AND WORKOUTS BOOST YOUR ENERGY. "Before Fit in 10, I was kind of weak, and now I have amazing endurance. There's no grandmom here, baby!"

◀ BEFORE

and drinking your breakfast for the next 4 weeks. Then, reality—often in the form of hunger, demanding schedules, pure exhaustion, or all three—hits, and boom: Your resolve falls apart like a wet paper towel.

It's a classic case of too much, too soon. Not only does it make you miserable, but it's also totally unnecessary. In fact, research shows that taking small steps toward a big goal isn't only easier and more sustainable—it's effective. According to a clinical review published in the *International Journal of Clinical Practice*,[11] when people with diabetes and cardiometabolic disorders made small diet or exercise changes that barely made a blip on their radar (like trimming 50 calories a day from their diet or walking a half-mile more each day), they saw significant weight loss and health improvements. What's more, they saw even greater benefit when they made a number of small changes together—just like you'll do, when you start doing one Fit in 10 routine a day and whipping up the simple yet delicious Fit in 10 meals.

"Big goals can be too overwhelming to tackle," says Dr. Sonya Lyubomirsky, professor of psychology at the University of California, Riverside. "Some of us will just procrastinate on them or give up altogether. Breaking up big goals into chunks, or baby steps, makes them seem more feasible and achievable."

Using the simple, 10-minutes-at-a-time approach was life changing for panelist Kimberlee Auerbach Berlin. When the 43-year-old thought about trying to lose the 60 pounds she'd gained with three pregnancies over the last 4 years, she felt hopeless. "It felt so daunting," says Berlin. "I thought I would have to stop eating and work out 2 hours a day. When you're busy, stressed, and sleep-deprived, you can't even imagine carving out that kind of time for yourself." But when Berlin started nurturing her body with 10-minute meals and workouts, she realized that this new, healthy lifestyle wasn't only doable—it was maintainable. "It made the impossible, possible," says Berlin, who dropped 14.5 pounds in 60 days. "The small, simple steps can really make a big difference."

Panelist Eileen Clark, 51, agrees and found that when she thought about trying to lose 20 pounds, she felt frustrated. "However," she says, "when I thought about losing 5 pounds at a time—and getting there with simple, 10-minute changes—it seemed much more manageable."

It Works at Any Stage of Your Life

No matter how many candles were on your last birthday cake or where you are on your health journey, embracing the 10-minute mind-set and purposefully applying it to your nutrition, exercise, and any other area of your life you want to improve will transform your life. Take Sarah M, a 33-year-old freelance consultant living and working in New York City, who lost 18 pounds on the Fit in 10 program. When she isn't putting in hours building her business, she's out with friends, often until 2 or 3 in the morning. Even though she was already active—she trained for triathalons and half marathons a few times a year—she struggled with her weight and needed a simple plan that would work with her on-the-go lifestyle. "Before learning how to eat clean, my diet was heavy on takeout and processed carbs," she said. "I'd end up eating sandwiches for three meals a day, like a fast-food egg sandwich for breakfast, a big deli sandwich for lunch, and a burger for dinner. Now, I know how to fuel my body without it having to take up a lot of my time."

Fit in 10 is also a saving grace for moms who are floundering trying to do it all or who currently don't have the time or freedom to work out like they used to before kids came along. "My husband is an assistant principal and is often out of the house before my daughter wakes up, so I'm primarily responsible for all of the parenting duties," says Ali McDowell. "Even though I'd try to work out three or four times a week, my schedule isn't always the same. When I have to make the 2-hour commute to my office, I have zero time to get to the gym," says McDowell. "Now, it doesn't matter if it's morning, noon, or night—I just tell my husband or daughter 'I'm going to go do my 10 minutes,' and they know what that means."

Finally, I've seen Fit in 10 click for women in their fifties and sixties who were struggling to find a way to offset the hormonal shift and weight creep of menopause while building strength and health for the second half of their life. When 52-year-old administrative assistant Janice Bishko found herself in a new romance after divorcing in 2014, she knew she needed a simple, sustainable way to curb relationship weight gain before it got out of hand. "We'd been dating for a little over a year and had gotten into a comfort zone," says Bishko, who lost 9 pounds and trimmed 4 inches off her middle in 8 weeks. "If I hadn't discovered Fit in 10, I'd never have lost the weight so easily. In the past, I'd try to get myself to do some sort of fitness regimen, but I never had the motivation or time. Ten minutes made it easy."

No matter your age, occupation, or what's going on in your life, Fit in 10 can work for you. You just have to commit to 10 minutes at a time and stick with it.

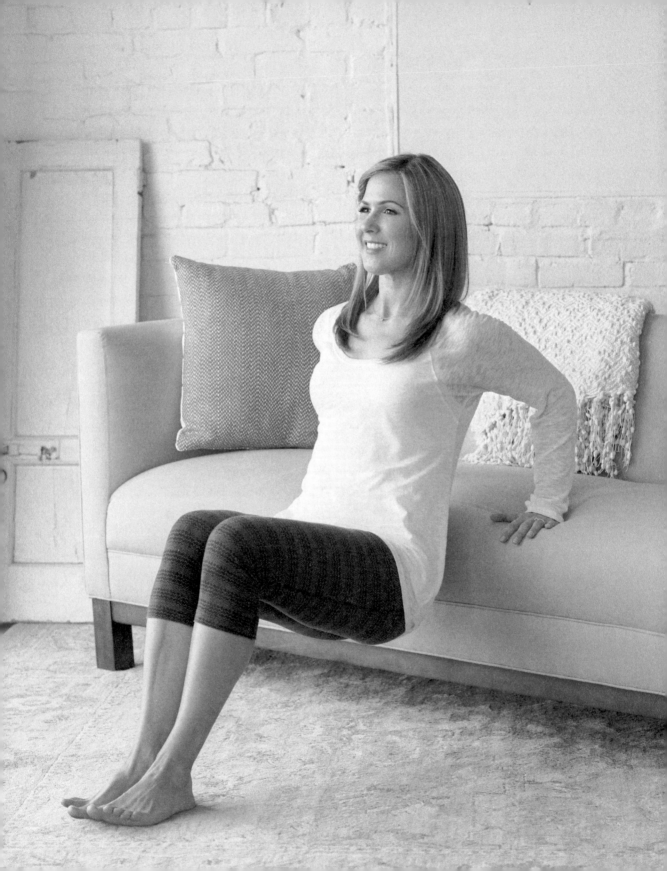

2

Take 10 to Look and Feel Your Best

"How am I ever going to fit it all in?" is a question I used to ask myself a lot before Fit in 10. Between family, work, a long commute, and keeping my house livable (I gave up on perfect a long time ago), there never seemed to be enough hours in the day. Before I knew it, I'd turn around and it would be 10 o'clock at night, and I hadn't gotten half of what I'd hope to accomplish crossed off my list.

Now, no matter how crazy my day, I know that I can take 10 minutes to strengthen and care for my body or squeeze in a little more of the things in life that give me true joy. That's what Fit in 10 is all about.

Hopefully by now you're excited to start your Fit in 10 journey, and this chapter is going to show you just how easy it is to incorporate into your current lifestyle. (Many women find it so unobtrusive that family and friends have no clue they've even started!) Whether you've been struggling to find the time to eat well and move more or you would rather spend more time doing other things, this program will help you lose stubborn weight, get back in shape simply, and create a life you love. In the next few pages, you'll discover how to nourish and strengthen your body in just minutes a day with our Fit in 10 formula, which has helped hundreds of women transform their bodies and feel and look years younger. You'll also learn how to optimize your day with 10-Minute Life Changers that'll do everything from boost your productivity and reduce your stress to enhance your relationships.

How the Fit in 10 Plan Works

Fit in 10: Slim & Strong—for Life! is based on cutting-edge research, but it doesn't require you to be a rocket scientist to do it—which is why it works so well. It simply takes a lot of what you already know you should be doing—eating clean and strength training regularly—and makes it so manageable and easy to implement that it's nearly impossible to fail.

Each day, you'll enjoy clean and delicious 10-minute meals and do one 10-minute toning routine. You'll also have the option to speed your transformation and enhance your life in other ways with the 10-Minute Life Changers found throughout this book. It's that simple!

While Fit in 10 is a lifestyle, not a diet, we've put together a 60-day program to help you jump-start your commitment to a healthy, active life. Research shows that it takes about that long to create new exercise and eating habits. After just 8 weeks, you'll have improved your health, toned and tightened your body, and made Fit in 10 a part of your daily life.

You'll learn more about each component in coming chapters, but here is a quick overview of the Fit in 10 pillars—plus, insider info on how to get the most out of the program.

The 10-Minute Meals

If you love good food as much as I do, get ready to enjoy every bite. These quick and delicious Fit in 10 recipes (all 85 of them) were developed at the Rodale Test Kitchen in Emmaus, Pennsylvania, and vetted by me, our test panelists, and their families. (Find them starting on page 161.) I know how hard it can be to put clean food on the table after a busy day (and what a challenge it can be to motivate yourself to cook a healthy meal), and that's why these meals are so fantastically simple. Many of the recipes require no more than 10 minutes in the kitchen, while others need just 10 minutes of "hands-on" time (so you'll chop, mix, and prep for 10 minutes or less, then pop the dish in the oven or turn on the slow cooker). This means that you'll be able to pick and choose meals depending on your schedule, your mood, and what you feel like eating that day.

But don't let their simplicity fool you. These meals are also incredibly tasty. Many of our test panelists couldn't believe these dishes were actually good for them—until the panelists started to notice how quickly their energy

The Fit in 10 success formula

10-minute meals
+
10-minute workouts
+
10-minute life changers

= Slim and Strong for Life!

rebounded and how easily the extra weight began to fall away.

That's because every breakfast, lunch, dinner, and snack has the perfect mix of hunger-staving lean protein, healthy fat, and nutrient-rich carbs to accelerate fat loss and optimize muscle building. The result: You'll lose weight while maximizing your metabolism and keeping your taste buds happy. Because the recipes are low in added sugar—an ingredient that increases inflammation—you may also notice a reduction in aches and pains (another perk our test panelists enjoyed).

So, how should you use them? Well, I love to have flexibility and choices, and I'm guessing you do, too. If your main goal for starting this

1O-MINUTE LIFE CHANGER
Tackle the Toughest Job First

Why is it that we tend to put off the jobs that need doing the most for as long as humanly possible? For me, sometimes that means avoiding writing an involved e-mail to a writer, having a difficult conversation with my partner, or even just dealing with unpleasant chores around the house, like going through that massive pile of mail. What happens? I waste precious mental energy worrying about the fact that I still need to do X and wind up feeling anxious and stressed knowing that it's still looming.

"Most people tend to put off a stressful or unpleasant task because they want to delay the unpleasantness as long as possible," says Peter Turla, time-management expert and president of the National Management Institute, a company that helps businesses develop a more productive and positive workforce. "The downside of doing this, however, is that we experience the unpleasantness anyway. Instead of simply dealing with the task when it's time to deal with it, we experience the mental tension and discomfort over and over again simply by thinking about it. This keeps our thoughts in a negative cycle that creates stress, a bad mood, and lowered productivity."

However, according to Turla, when you tackle a job or task right away—instead of putting it off as long as humanly possible—you tend to work with a clearer mind, you're more relaxed, and you're better able to focus. Plus, you save all of the energy you would have wasted worrying about it.

So the next time you find yourself postponing the inevitable, apply the Fit in 10 mentality and take 10 minutes to just deal with whatever it is, right now. I've found that 99 percent of the time the thing that I was so worried about is never as unpleasant as my monkey brain was making it out to be. Once it's done, I'm happier and more productive. Now, it's your turn to try it.

plan is to lose weight, then start by following the 10-Day Clean-Eating Jump Start that begins on page 151. This will show you how to mix and match the Fit in 10 recipes so that you stay within an ideal calorie range for weight loss. Otherwise, browse through the meals and choose the ones that sound best to you or that work for your diet limitations. In whatever way you choose to use them, the Fit in 10 meals make eating clean fast and enjoyable—even on the busiest of days.

The 10-Minute Workouts

It's kind of amazing when you realize how easy it is to get strong and lean with the Fit in 10 routines. Right at home, and whenever you please. They're so doable that I, and many of our test panelists, often do them in our pajamas right before hopping into the shower in the morning or at the end of a long day.

I worked with my friend and trainer Larysa DiDio to design the workouts. Each of the twelve 10-minute routines in this book includes a careful mix of metabolism-revving sculpting moves that can be modified for every fitness level. Another great perk: They'll also up your energy and help you build lean, beautiful muscle. The more muscle mass you have, the easier it is to maintain a healthy weight, the better your clothes fit, and the easier it is to move effortlessly throughout life with energy and fewer aches and pains.

Just like the Fit in 10 recipes, the Fit in 10 routines are all about choices. The workouts are divided into four Tone Zones—Upper Body, Lower Body, Belly, and Total Body—so you can mix and match the routines depending on your goals or energy levels. Many of our test panelists loved that they could flip to whichever body part they wanted to tone that day—whether it was their belly, butt, or arms—and feel the burn in their target area in just 10 minutes.

However, if you're looking to tone every inch while you lose weight and build strength, I suggest that you follow the 60-day plan outlined on page 42. Each day you'll do a different routine to maximize your results. As you get stronger, you always have the option to stack the workouts and do two or more on the same day. If you're just starting out or have struggled to stay consistent with exercise in the past, stick to the plan and do just one 10-minute routine each day. You'll be surprised by how quickly your body changes when you commit to 10 minutes a day. Pick the option that works best for you and your body, go slow, and get ready to watch your strength, energy, and body transform.

The 10-Minute Life Changers

Once I realized how effective 10 minutes of smart strength training was for toning my body, I started to wonder what would happen if I applied the 10-minute mentality to other areas of my life. I noticed that embracing the power of 10 left me feeling more calm, focused,

Christine Szpynda

"Overworked and over-booked" is how Christine Szpynda described her life when she signed up for the *Fit in 10: Slim & Strong–for Life!* program. The 45-year-old wife and mother of three was juggling a career as an executive director at a large financial services company with a busy home life. Her nonstop schedule–combined with the fact that her weight had steadily been creeping up since she'd hit her forties–left her feeling tired all the time. The evening run she'd done on and off for years had been "off" for longer than she'd like to admit, thanks to her achy knees, and she needed a simple routine she could do in the morning before the craziness of her day started. "My days only seemed to get busier as they went on, which made finding the time to exercise really challenging," she says. "I'd tell myself I'd start working out on Monday and then it would be Wednesday and I still hadn't done anything. It was this big, depressing cycle."

When Christine started using the Fit in 10 program, she discovered that she didn't have to work out for an hour at a time to see results. "I felt a difference right away," she says. "I thought, *Wow, I can work out for 10 minutes before I leave the house to catch my train to work, and even if I do nothing active the rest of the day, I can feel proud that I got a workout in.* It felt so positive and made

AGE:	**45**
POUNDS LOST:	**16**
INCHES LOST:	**21.75**

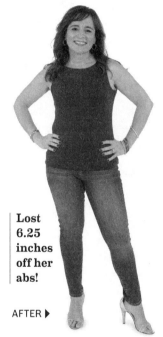

Lost 6.25 inches off her abs!

AFTER ▶

me feel like I was moving in the right direction."

Even though her kitchen was in the middle of a renovation and Christine wasn't able to make as many of the Fit in 10 recipes as she would have liked, she cleaned up her diet and started trading processed carbs like pizza and cookies for salads and salmon. "There were plenty of healthy choices I could make when I went out to eat," she says. "I didn't feel like I was on a diet at all."

Within a few weeks, Christine started to notice changes in her body. Her belly started to shrink and she had to start pulling her "skinny" clothes out from storage. "I can go shopping in my closet again," she laughs. "Things that used to be tight on me are suddenly loose. I feel like my old self again. Fit in 10 taught me that getting and staying in shape is really just about three things: knowledge, commitment, and consistency."

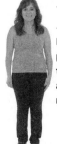

Why Christine Loves Fit in 10

IT GIVES YOU A DOABLE PLAN. "I was at a point in my life where I wanted and needed to make a change, but I was kind of frozen and I didn't know what to do. Fit in 10 showed me exactly how to live the life I wanted."

◀ BEFORE

and productive—and less overwhelmed. Even though my life wasn't less busy, I was finally doing more of the things that mattered to me and getting some of those stressful "should dos" out of the way much sooner than normal.

Once you realize how much of an impact 10 minutes can make on your health and body, you'll want to apply the 10-minute fix to other areas of your life, too. That's why you'll find 10-Minute Life Changers throughout this book and also in the *Fit in 10 Journal*.

In the first week or two, you may want to focus on getting the nutrition and fitness down—and that's totally fine. However, once you become more comfortable with the 10-minute meals and workouts, start experimenting with adding at least one new 10-Minute Life Changer to your routine each week. They're optional, but doing them will help you have better success on the plan. Plus, they're fun and easy. You'll be surprised at how much of a difference these little 10-minute tweaks can make.

How to Get the Most out of the Plan

Research shows that up to two-thirds of dieters regain the pounds they lost and then some within a few years.[1] What does work: Cultivating a clean-eating and active lifestyle that feels so good that it naturally becomes your baseline. When people make lifestyle changes they can maintain, like eating healthier foods and moving more, they're more likely to lose weight and keep it off.[2]

Long after the first 60 days are over, you'll find yourself continuing to enjoy the Fit in 10 lifestyle. You'll find an entire chapter about how to eat clean in the real world (see page 131). You'll learn how to make smart choices at the grocery store, at restaurants, and when you're traveling. You'll also discover simple tips to shorten the amount of time you spend in the kitchen. While I have no doubt that you'll enjoy the Fit in 10 meals included in this book, understanding the basics of clean eating will also give you the freedom to be creative when you cook.

In order to help you start off right and to kick-start your weight loss, follow the 60-day nutrition and toning plan outlined in the next few chapters and chart your progress in a daily journal.

After you complete the 60-day plan, you may find that you feel so good on Fit in 10 that you want to start the plan over again to keep working toward your goals (as did many of our test panelists). If that's the case, go for it! If you want to be a bit more lax after completing the 60-day plan, yet maintain your results, keep this book on hand as a guide to a healthier, happier life and aim to follow the Fit in 10 principles at least 80 percent of the time. Do this, and I promise you that you will enjoy an energized life and a stronger, healthier body. When you get off track, as we all do from time to time, pick up this book to rekindle your motivation and consider following the 60-day program again to hit your reset button and maintain a healthy weight.

Make Sure to Journal

Think of your journal like your own personal Fit in 10 coach: It will help you stay motivated and on track for the next 60 days. Jot down your starting stats (like your weight and measurements). As the days pass, you will be able to monitor your progress along the way. Each day, take note of your mood, workouts, water intake, and, of course, your Fit in 10 meals. Research shows that keeping a food diary can double your weight loss. In fact, in a study of nearly 1,700 participants, those who tracked their meals lost twice as much weight as those who kept no records.[3]

Plus, our test panelists found a journal to be super useful and fun. "My journal definitely kept me on track," says Janice Bishko. "I loved the sense of accomplishment I felt every time I checked off a workout or a glass of water."

YOUR BUSY LIFE IN NUMBERS

Feel like there are never enough hours in the day? You're not the only one. Out of 100 women surveyed . . .

✳ **75 PERCENT** feel that it's nearly impossible to get in or stay in shape when life gets busy.

✳ **68 PERCENT** say that trying to lose weight and keep it off has made them feel crazy and out of control at some point in their life.

✳ Due to their busy schedules, **26 PERCENT** estimate they've gained 5 to 10 pounds; 24 percent estimate they've gained 10 to 20 pounds; 16 percent estimate they've gained 20 to 30 pounds; and 15 percent estimate they've gained 30 or more pounds.

✳ **48 PERCENT** say they have tried numerous diet and exercise programs but have quit when they became too time consuming to maintain.

✳ **78 PERCENT** say putting their body's needs last has negatively impacted their confidence.

> The good news? Almost 90 PERCENT say they could easily find 10 minutes in their day to exercise or make a healthy meal. Which means there's no excuse not to get Fit in 10!

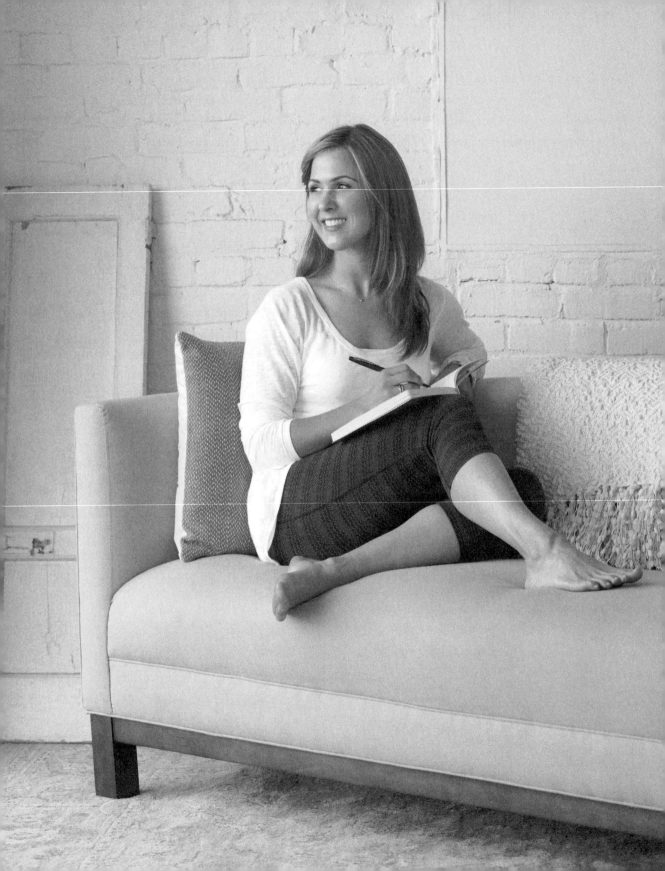

3

Fit in 10
Success Strategies

Now that you know the Fit in 10 formula for creating the body and life that you want, it's time to talk about the other half of the winning equation: you! Even though Fit in 10 makes getting and staying in shape amazingly simple, there are still going to be times when you momentarily forget your blessings and feel grumbly and resistant to squeezing in a workout or making a quick trip to the grocery store. I've been a morning exerciser for years, and there's still a tug-of-war that goes on inside my head when the alarm blares and I have to decide if I'm going to sleep for a few more precious minutes or get up and move my body. I've learned that it's the way I talk to myself in those decisive moments that determines whether I move forward or stay stuck.

"The other part is mental," agrees Tanya Szozda-Komaniecki, 43, who lost 6 pounds on the Fit in 10 program. "Whenever I started to feel down on myself or a little unmotivated, I'd repeat the mantra, 'What you feed the body, you feed the soul.'" Anytime she thought of that affirmation, Szozda-Komaniecki felt inspired to give herself only good stuff, both through healthy movement and healthy food. "It really encouraged me to stay focused on the end goal," she says.

These little mental tricks make all the difference, which is why you'll find the next few pages filled with science-backed ways to help make Fit in 10 even easier. So for the mornings when you hit the snooze button too many times, the afternoons when your energy is low and your temper is short, and those nights when your partner suggests ordering pizza and it sounds so freakin' good, keep these success strategies in mind.

Stay Clear about Why You're Doing This

Almost anyone who loses weight and keeps it off can tell you about the "aha moment" that motivated her to transform her life and body. That split second when she decided she'd had enough, when the light switch of determination was flicked on inside her heart and nothing was going to stop her. For Anne Marie Russo, it was buying a one-piece swimsuit after a lifetime of wearing bikinis (see her story on page 129). For Sarah M., it was finishing a half marathon 45 minutes after her friends (see her story on page 45). And for me, it was seeing a photo of my 12-year-old self that was taken at my cousin's bar mitzvah party.

In order to understand why this photo carried such impact, you first need a little insight into the psyche of a sixth-grader. In my mind, my cousin's initiation into manhood was my first chance to go to a real-deal party, and I was amped about it. My hair was curled, I was wearing a pretty new dress, and I'd swiped mascara and lip gloss from my mom's makeup bag. I felt beautiful, and I spent that entire eve-

ning dancing with the cute boys and hamming it up for anyone who would point the camera my way. Then, a few weeks later, I saw the photos and my heart crumpled. Who *was* that girl in my party dress, the heavy one with the round face and glasses? She couldn't possibly be me, could she? I'd had this image of what I'd looked like that night in my mind, and it wasn't matching up with the reality of what had been captured on film.

Looking back now, I want to tell 12-year-old me that I *was* beautiful that day, just as I was. But 22 years ago that disconnect between whom I knew myself to be on the inside and whom I saw on the outside saddened me. It wasn't just that I wanted to lose weight or fit into smaller jeans. It went far deeper than that. I wanted to feel like *me*. I had a sudden, overwhelming desire to unearth the person I actually was: the girl who was hiding beneath the extra weight.

A few weeks later, a gym teacher randomly popped in a Richard Simmons's *Sweatin' to the Oldies* DVD and (nerd alert) . . . I freakin' loved it. This wasn't brutal or painful exercise. This was fun. I went home, begged my mom for my own copy, and spent the rest of the year and following summer dancing in my living room. By the beginning of seventh grade, people told me I looked like a new person. I finally felt like myself.

The thing is, seeing that photo wasn't the first time that I might have realized that my extra weight wasn't serving me. There had been numerous other opportunities that could have served as my aha moment. Kids had said mean things. My pediatrician had talked over my head to my mom, more than once, letting her know I needed to "slim down." Our fridge was filled with nothing but healthy snacks. The reason that photo changed my life was because I was ready, and I had found a meaningful reason to make a change.

If you're reading this, I hope that you've found the intention that will inspire you to create the life you want. If not, take a few minutes to think about what's truly driving you to start this program and try to go beyond the numbers on the scale or the standard, two-dimensional desire to "be thin." That's not to say that some of what I'll call "surface intention" isn't important. It's not fun feeling as though nothing in your closet fits you, or that every summer you won't leave the house in a tank top without grabbing a cardigan. But the truth is, our bodies change, and especially as we age, many of us are no longer deeply motivated by the goal of fitting into skinny jeans. In fact, according to a 2013 study published in the journal *Obesity*,[1] women ages 36 to 50 were more likely to cite health than appearance as a motivator for weight loss compared to younger adults. And that change in perspective could actually help you lose weight and keep it off more easily. Research also shows that people who get in shape to improve their health or to redirect course after a medical scare lose more weight and are able to keep it off longer than people who are motivated by appearance alone. [2]

So start by thinking about how you want to feel instead of just how you want to look. Do you want to be healthy, strong, energetic, and youthful? Whatever it is, jot it down. Then go deeper by asking yourself what you want your future to look like. Fit in 10 test panelist Lori Lowell envisioned the second half of her life as

10-MINUTE LIFE CHANGER
Clutter-Proof Your Kitchen

If your house is anything like mine, there are days when the kitchen counter seems to be a catchall for everything from dirty dishes to the day's mail. However, regularly taking just 10 minutes to tidy up the space could make a big difference in your waistline. Women ate nearly 40 percent more cookies when they were in a chaotic kitchen and feeling out of control than when they were in an organized, clutter-free space, according to research from the Cornell University Food and Brand Lab.[3] Research also shows that putting snack food out of sight can cut down mindless munching by 50 percent.[4] So put 10 minutes on the kitchen timer and clear off those counters, put away the dishes, and tuck your kids' cereal boxes and snack food into cabinets where they will be out of sight and out of mind.

an active one. "At 59, I'm no longer 'bikini body' material, but I do want to be fit," says Lowell. "I found that my joints were starting to ache and that I was slowing down and feeling more fatigued. I decided to start this program because I wanted to be stronger. When I'm 80, I want to be the little old lady that's still getting out there."

In the long run, building your intention on a strong foundation will help you stay motivated, especially on those days when your willpower is tested.

The Only Person You Can Change Is *You*

Sometimes we're so excited to start our health journey that we expect everyone around us to join in and come along for the ride. When that works, it's awesome. After all, it's motivating when your partner, kids, coworkers, or friends cheer you along, and it's easier to stay on track when you're all eating the same clean foods.

Unfortunately, that doesn't always happen. Sometimes our "support circle" can be anything *but* supportive when it comes to weight loss, according to a 2014 published in the *Journal of Human Nutrition and Dietetics*.[5] Researchers asked 23 women who had successfully completed an 18-week weight loss program to answer open-ended questions about the hurdles they encountered losing weight and trying to keep it off—and their answers were pretty surprising. While some women found their

friends and family to be helpful and encouraging, the majority of the group felt just the opposite. The study participants said that it wasn't unusual for friends, family, and coworkers to tempt them with high-calorie junk foods or make unhelpful comments regarding their new healthy eating habits, especially at family meals, social gatherings, or restaurants. Comments like "You don't need to lose weight"; "You're having a salad again today?"; and "Go ahead and eat dessert, you deserve it" were reported. While the study participants considered such comments to be unintentional forms of diet sabotage, they still found them to make sticking to their healthy habits more difficult.

It can be especially challenging when a family member is resistant. A 2015 study published in the journal *Obesity*[6] found that dieters who experience lack of, or inconsistent, support at home were more likely to struggle with weight loss and regain the pounds they'd lost within 2 years. Additionally, several studies indicate that accommodating family members' food preferences made it harder for women to eat healthy and manage their weight.

That's why it's vital to stay focused on your intention and to remember that you can only control your own behaviors. Often, when you stick to your plan, those around you will start to follow suit. For instance, when my husband and I started living together, we ate completely differently. His diet was full of frozen pizzas, sugary cereals, and other processed foods. At first,

Linda Cohen

When Linda Cohen saw a Facebook post announcing that *Prevention* was looking for busy women like her to test the new *Fit in 10: Slim & Strong–for Life!* plan, she knew she had to apply. The program appealed to the stay-at-home mom of two teens–a 16-year-old daughter and 14-year-old son–for multiple reasons. "First, I really liked that it talked about becoming lean and strong instead of skinny," says Linda. "Being strong is really important to me. In fact, when my kids were little, they would ask why I was going to the gym and I often said it was so that I could be strong enough to pick them up and take care of them."

Linda also liked the idea of losing the 10 pounds that had slowly crept on over the last few years. Even though she enjoyed being active and consistently went to boot camp and yoga a few times a week or biked with her family on the weekends, her metabolism seemed to be slowing down. She hadn't changed her habits or schedule, but her clothes were getting tighter, especially around the middle.

When Linda started following the Fit in 10 meal plan and doing the extra 10 minutes of exercise each day, she was amazed at how quickly she started to see and feel a difference. "One of the best parts of the Fit in 10 program was the 10-Day Clean-Eating Jump Start because all the

AGE:	44
POUNDS LOST:	7
INCHES LOST:	17

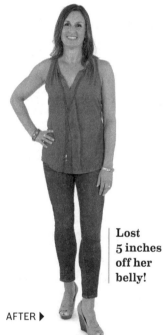

Lost 5 inches off her belly!

AFTER ▶

work was done," says Linda. "I knew I was getting all of the protein and calories I needed, and I knew that all my food groups were covered. It was a really easy way to literally jump-start the weight loss. It was terrific."

Linda also found adding the extra 10 minutes to her routine worked best if she did it first thing each morning. "If I waited until the end of the day, then it seemed like more of a chore for me," she says. "But doing the exercises first thing in the morning made it just part of my waking up, and I loved that."

By the end of the plan, Linda could see and feel a difference in her waist. "Everything is more comfortable and I don't feel like I need to hide my belly anymore," she says. "I can tuck in my shirts, and I was even confident enough to wear a two-piece swimsuit in public for the first time in years this summer. It helped me take my body to the next level and see the results I wanted."

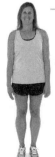

Why Linda Loves Fit in 10

IT TONES EVERY ZONE. "I loved that the workouts were sectioned by upper body, lower body, belly, and total body. It was nice to mix and match them if I was feeling really strong and wanted to add 10 minutes of belly or arms."

◀ BEFORE

I encouraged him to go clean, but he wasn't having it. So instead of pressing the issue, I often would prepare a clean meal for myself and let him do his own thing. Over time, though, he began to try more of the healthier foods I cooked and, to his surprise, started to enjoy them. Eventually, when I announced I was making chicken and sweet potatoes or spaghetti squash and meat sauce for dinner, he'd say, "Sounds good. I'll have it, too."

Find Your Cheerleaders

If your family isn't giving you the support you need, it's important to find a support network you can count on to keep you motivated. Research shows that accountability and support from others increases weight loss and weight loss maintenance in dieters, according to a 2014 study published in the journal *Obesity*.[7] "My biggest challenge is living alone and not having someone to keep me accountable," agrees 60-year-old test panelist Nancy A. Shenker. "So I decided to tell my interns at work that I was doing the program. They started asking me a lot of questions about what I was doing, which helped keep me on track." Shenker also posted on Facebook that she was looking for a Fit in 10 workout buddy who could meet up with her once a week. Merlyn Joseph, 53, another Fit in 10 test panelist, quickly agreed to join her. "Knowing I was going to work out with a friend gave me something to look forward to," says Shenker. So don't be afraid to reach out to online friends, neighbors, or coworkers. Not only will you most likely see better results, but you'll have more fun, too.

Be Smart about the Scale

We've all been there: standing naked, vulnerable, and full of angst in front of that torturous little device that sits on the bathroom floor. No matter how you try to get around it—holding your breath, stepping on super gently, holding on to the sink with one hand—the scale instantly reveals *the number*. If it's in the zone you want, well, then life is good. If not, well . . . watch out. In my career as a health and fitness editor, I've yet to meet a woman who truly enjoys getting on the scale. For most us, it's about as pleasant as getting a tooth filled.

For a long time, I felt the same way. In fact, in high school, my friend and I had a joke about the "scale conspiracy." We believed that no matter what our scales at home said, the scale at the doctor's office weighed us at least 10 pounds heavier. Just to, you know, mess with us. It was our way of making fun of the numbers and not allowing them to bother us so much.

While I believe that our self-worth and confidence should have nothing to do with the scale (we are all so much more than a number), I have learned over the years that it can be a valuable tool for weight loss. In fact, a study of 91 overweight adults in the *Journal of the Academy of Nutrition and Dietetics* found that those who weighed themselves daily lost more weight compared to those who did it weekly or not at all.[8] It turns out that daily weigh-ins can act as a sort of a reset button that reminds you of your goal and encourages you to stick with your healthy eating and exercise habits.

However, daily monitoring may only be effective for "certain adults," according to a study by Cornell University researchers.[9] If you're prone to obsessive behavior, have ever struggled with disordered eating, or just feel like your day is completely ruined after stepping on the scale, regular weigh-ins may actually be counterproductive in your weight loss journey.[10] If this sounds like you, then watch for other signs about how well you're taking care of your body, including how your clothes are fitting, how well you're sleeping, and what your energy levels are like.

Don't Let One Poor Choice Derail You

One of the reasons that diets don't work is that diet plans have hard-and-fast rules. So when the inevitable happens and we—*gasp*—put something in our mouths that was not part of the program, we can beat ourselves up. Even worse, we often go straight to the conclusion that we might as well just give up.

We rarely act this childish in other areas of our lives, do we? If a child ruins a trip to Target with a tantrum, do we say, "Oh, well, now this whole parenting thing is ruined. Let's just call it off. I'll start over with the next kid." Or if we have a squabble with a partner, do we head straight to the courthouse for a divorce? Hopefully not.

"Well," you might be thinking, "that's a silly comparison. After all, a diet is transient; parenting and partnership are for life. How can you compare?"

True, a diet isn't forever. But clean eating is a lifestyle, not a diet, and something that I will happily follow for the rest of my life—and hopefully you will, too. There will be "slipups" and "bad days." That's okay! That's life. But instead of allowing those mistakes to snowball into processed-food chaos, try to adopt a calm manner about it. You are in this for the long game. You are now a professional clean eater. Go right back to clean at the next meal or snack. Do this, and you will not only lose weight, but you'll keep it off. In fact, dieters who adopted this "fresh slate" mentality lost more weight over 18 weeks than dieters who weren't able shake off small setbacks, according to a 2014 study published in the *Journal of Human Nutrition and Dietetics*.[11]

MINUTES TO MINDFULNESS

You don't need start meditating for hours every day. You can start to strengthen your mind-body connection and practice mindfulness simply by taking your attention to your breath. Try it now: Allow yourself to feel your chest rise and fall. Notice if your breath is quick or shallow and then start to deepen your breath, aiming for about 4 counts as you inhale and 4 counts as you exhale. Then, start to notice the other sensations in and around your body. What can you feel, hear, smell, or touch? Allow all of these sensations to pull you out of your mind and into your body and the present moment. Practice this simple technique for a few minutes each day, and anytime your thoughts feel chaotic. Over time, you'll strengthen your mindfulness muscle and be more likely to hear what your body is trying to tell you.

Tune In to Your Body

We're often so distracted by the thoughts and to-dos whirling around inside our heads that we barely notice what's happening in the present moment. Instead, we worry about what's coming up in the future or what went wrong in the past. The result: We totally miss the opportunity to live in the now, which can cause us to overlook some important messages about our health and body.

In fact, learning to cultivate this presence, or mindfulness, won't just bring you a little more peace and calm—new research shows that it could also help you slim down. People who live in the moment tend to have less body fat, especially around the belly, according to a study published in the *International Journal of Behavioral Medicine*.[12] Researchers at Brown University measured the body composition and mindfulness disposition of 400 individuals and found that people with low levels of mindfulness were 34 percent more likely to be obese and carried more fat around their bellies compared to study participants that spent less time on automatic pilot. According to the researchers, people who are more mindful are more aware of how food and exercise affect their bodies and therefore make healthier choices based on how they feel. So, for example, when you're aware of how you feel in the present moment, you're less likely to eat past the point of fullness or to miss signs that your body would feel a lot better if you got off the couch and went for a walk.[13]

Plan Ahead for Crazy Days

You wouldn't tackle an important project at work without a strategy, right? Well, formulating a plan for how you'll stick to your Fit in 10 plan on a day-to-day basis will increase your chances of success. Research shows that women who planned their meals and exercise in advance have greater success with weight loss and keeping it off than women who were less organized.[14]

"If I didn't preplan, I would never make it!" says Tanya Szozda-Komaniecki. "On Sundays, I'll put together some extra parfaits and salads that I can grab for breakfast and lunch during the week. I'll also make kale chips for snacks and stick them in zipper bags so I can grab and go." (For more ideas on how to prep food for the week ahead, turn to page 142.)

Determining when you'll do your Fit in 10 routine will also go a long way in making sure it actually happens. Will you work out first thing in the morning, on your lunch break, or after the kids are in bed for the evening? "I always do a Fit in 10 routine in the morning before work," says Eileen Clark, 51. "It sets my tone for the day and then I have no excuse as to why I didn't get it done." So find the best time for you and then stick with it.

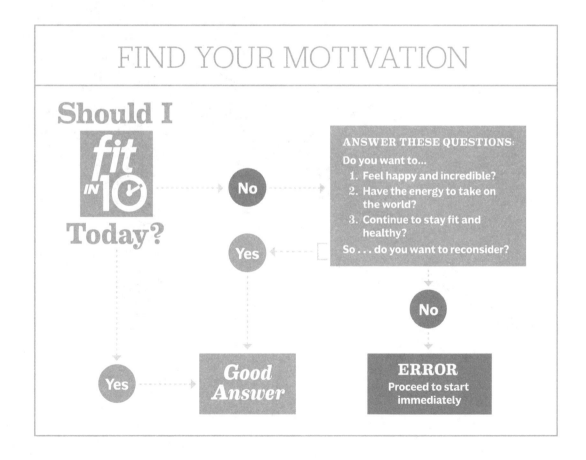

FIND YOUR MOTIVATION

Should I *fit IN 10* **Today?**

No

Yes

ANSWER THESE QUESTIONS:
Do you want to...
1. Feel happy and incredible?
2. Have the energy to take on the world?
3. Continue to stay fit and healthy?

So . . . do you want to reconsider?

No

Yes

Good Answer

ERROR
Proceed to start immediately

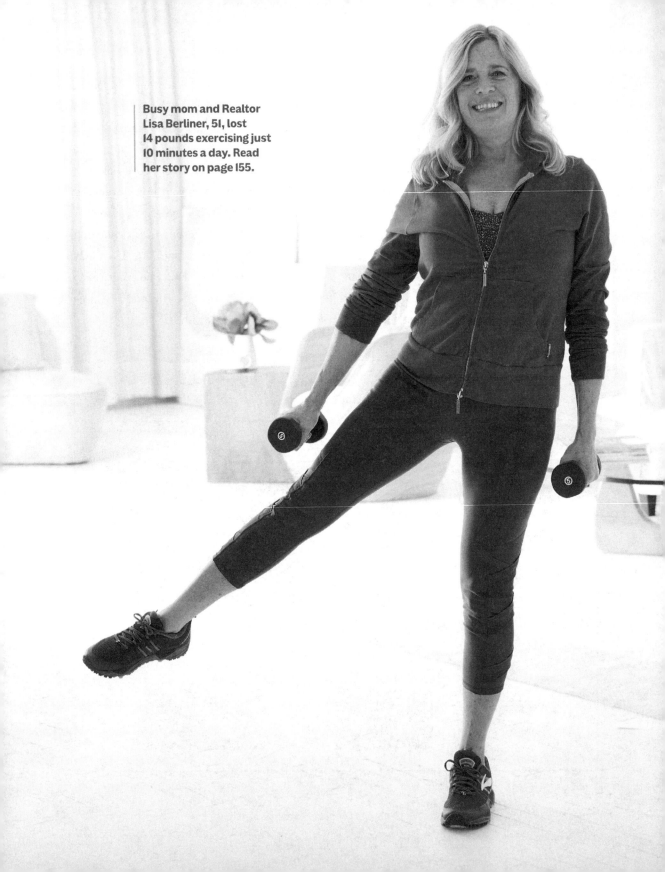

Busy mom and Realtor
Lisa Berliner, 51, lost
14 pounds exercising just
10 minutes a day. Read
her story on page 155.

4

Slimmer, Stronger–Simply

How do you want to live the second half of your life? When I posed this question to our *Fit in 10: Slim & Strong—for Life!* test panel, they had a lot to say. They talked about wanting to feel healthy and young for as long as possible. To wake up every day energized and free of pain, capable of taking care of themselves and their families. To be fit, and not frail, so they could play with their kids and grandkids, and plan the adventures and take the trips they always imagined taking. Most of all, they wanted to feel lean and strong and empowered in their bodies. Not to fit anyone else's "ideal" body type, but for themselves.

I couldn't agree with their sentiments more. We need to be strong physically and mentally. Strength is freedom. Strength is power. Strength is beautiful. And being able to achieve all of the above in less time than it takes to clean up dinner? Well, that's awesome.

"Often people think they need to commit to 60 minutes at the gym, then feel overwhelmed and never get started," says Jordan Metzl, MD, a sports medicine physician at the Hospital for Special Surgery in New York City. "But even as little as 10 minutes of strength training a day can make a big difference in muscle strength and your overall health and fitness." That's the beauty of the Fit in 10 toning plan: It makes strength training so easy, doable, and fun that it naturally becomes a way of life.

Transform Your Body and Health

One of the best parts about the Fit in 10 routines is that they're *only* 10 minutes—as soon as they start to feel really challenging, they're over and you can get on with your day. But that little workout does some heavy lifting. Here are just a few of the ways picking up those weights daily will help you lose pounds and get your best self back.

Rekindle Your Metabolism

While genetics and gender certainly influence how many calories your body burns in a day, the Fit in 10 routines will stoke your body's energy-burning fire in multiple ways by helping you rebuild lean muscle. Starting at age 30, we begin to lose about a half a pound of the metabolism-revving tissue each year—and by midlife, the rate doubles. "The average sedentary woman may have lost nearly 15 pounds of muscle by the time she reaches her late fifties, a change that could cause her to gain nearly the same amount in body fat," says strength-training expert Wayne Westcott, PhD. That's a terrifying stat, when you consider that your muscle influences everything from how good you look in your jeans to how well you fend off disease. And the more lean mass you lose, the more your metabolism puts on the brakes.

Thankfully, it's never too late to start strength training. Research shows that women of all ages can revive youthful, metabolically active muscle when they pick up the weights. "When you do resistance training, it causes a degree of microtrauma, or tiny tears, to the muscle tissue," says Dr. Westcott. "Over the next 48 to 72 hours, your body remodels and heals that tissue with amino acids, making it stronger—or, if you're just starting out and need to gain muscle mass, the muscle slowly grows." This throws coals onto your metabolism's calorie-burning fire in two ways: First, the more muscle you build, the more calories you'll burn each day. Second, the rebuilding process itself requires extra energy, boosting your daily calorie burn by 5 percent to 9 percent.

Additionally, because the Fit in 10 routines keep you moving from one exercise to the next with little rest in between, you'll score another metabolic boost. "Taking only a brief break after each exercise burns extra calories and accelerates metabolism more than waiting the standard 60 to 90 seconds between sets," says Dr. Westcott.

Burn Off Belly Fat

Research shows that lifting weights can make a big difference in the size of your waist. When sedentary, postmenopausal women did two full-body strength-training sessions a week, they significantly reduced their body fat and waist circumference in just 6 weeks. They also increased their arm and leg strength while simultaneously reducing their resting heart rate, blood pressure, and blood sugar.[1]

Alternating between bursts of more intense exercise like squat jumps and more moderate ones like biceps curls (as you do in many of the Fit in 10 routines) helps you crush belly fat even faster. "This type of interval training elevates neurohormones, particularly epinephrine," says exercise physiologist Michele Olson, PhD, professor of exercise science at Auburn University Montgomery in Montgomery, Alabama. "Epinephrine has to rise markedly during high-intensity interval training in order to increase heart rate to the appropriate level. Additionally, epinephrine has also been found to increase the release of fat from the fat cells." So the harder you push, the more overall body fat you'll burn and the firmer and flatter your belly will look.

Reduce Aches and Pains

When you're uncomfortable in your body, it's really difficult to enjoy life. And while the Fit in 10 routines may make you feel *momentarily* uncomfortable by increasing your body temperature and causing your muscles to burn, those few minutes of unease can gain you years of fewer aches and pains. When women and men aged 55 years or older with knee pain performed a simple, at-home strength-training routine three times a week, they reported a 43 percent decrease in pain and a 44 percent increase in ease of movement after 4 months, according to a study published in the *Journal of Rheumatology.*[2]

Additionally, weight training has been shown to reduce stiffness and discomfort from chronic nonspecific low-back pain.[3] "Since

starting Fit in 10, I've had a huge reduction in back pain," says 52-year-old Janice Bishko. "I used to be so stiff and achy in the morning that I had trouble getting out of bed. Now, it's much easier to move around."

Fend Off Disease and Stay Mentally Sharp

Research shows that muscle is a very important tissue, and it's not just about how much you have—it's what's inside it that matters most. Metabolically active muscle—the kind that's free of harmful fat and teeming with mitochondria, the

LIFTING LINGO

Rep: This is shorthand for "repetition." So "one rep" simply means one complete motion of the exercise. If you're supposed to do 10 reps of a squat, for example, that just means you should do 10 squats.

Set: A set is a group of consecutive reps performed back-to-back without rest. So, for example, if you do 10 reps of a squat, that would be one set. If you rest and then do another 10 reps, then you would have done two sets. Sets are often measured by a number of prescribed reps, but they can also be measured by time. So for instance, you could do three sets of 30-second sets. This means that you'll do as many reps as possible with good form within that 30-second time frame, take a rest, and then repeat the 30 seconds of work two more times.

metabolism-boosting powerhouses within cells—has a profound influence on everything from your weight to your energy levels to your risks of diabetes and heart disease. Even your chances of surviving a hospital stay or beating cancer are affected by the health of your muscle.[4]

Regular strength training can help keep your muscles strong and youthful by helping the tissue stay lean. The less you move, the easier it is for fat to infiltrate your muscle, which makes your body less responsive to insulin, thereby making it easier to gain weight and harder to lose it. All of which increases your risk for diabetes.

Additionally, research shows that women who pick up the weights are more likely to stay mentally sharp. When researchers at the University of British Columbia monitored the effects of resistance training on seniors with mild cognitive impairment, they found that just 6 months of simple weight training improved executive cognitive functions, such as attention, memory, problem solving, and decision making.[5]

Tone Every Zone

Whether you want to build your butt, firm and flatten your abs, or lose the arm jiggle, the Fit in 10 routines will help you do it quickly. Unlike many traditional fitness programs that require you to do the same routine over and over, you'll rotate through 12 different workouts that will fight boredom while firming and strengthening every inch of your body. Each routine falls under one of four key Tone Zones—Upper Body, Lower Body, Belly, and Total Body—to ensure you'll shed fat and define every muscle in just 10 minutes a day. When you follow the toning plan that starts on page 42, you'll sculpt and strengthen your entire body while really zeroing in on common trouble spots, like abs and arms.

Get Slim and Strong for Life

Ready to get toned and energized in just 10 minutes a day? Before you get started with the 60-day toning plan on page 42, take a few minutes to read this section for tips and tricks that'll help you start strong and speed your results.

What Do You Need?

Honestly, not much. Very little equipment is required to tone in 10, and if you're just getting back to exercise, you'll feel and see a difference with nothing more than your own body weight. You'll accelerate your results and enjoyment of the plan, however, when you incorporate the following tools.

RESISTANCE BAND LOOPS. These stretchy bands easily slip around your ankles, thighs, and wrists to help you target hard-to-tone zones, like the hips, butt, thighs, and upper arms. Because the band places resistance on your muscles in multiple directions, you'll quickly start to feel your deepest muscles engage without placing a lot of stress on your joints. Another bonus: The bands are super light and fit easily into your purse or suitcase, so you can take them with you for on-the-go toning. Many of our test panelists took the bands with them on work trips, to the beach, even camping.

Choose a resistance level that allows you to perform as many reps as possible during each set with correct form. If you easily finish the set without feeling challenged, use a thicker band that offers more resistance. If you find that you're struggling to perform the full range of motion of the exercise, opt for a lighter resistance band. You may find that you'll need higher resistance for moves that activate your larger muscle groups (like the hips, butt, and thighs) and lighter resistance for exercises that challenge smaller muscle groups (like your biceps and triceps).

HAND WEIGHTS. In addition to the toning bands, you'll be using hand weights to build a strong, lean body. Ideally, you'll have three or four sets of dumbbells of varying weights (say, 5-, 8-, 10-, and 12-pound dumbbells) so you can add and decrease the resistance as needed. In the beginning—especially as you learn the exercises—you may feel best with 5- to 8-pound weights. As you progress, however, don't be afraid to challenge yourself. Increase your weight as soon as you can complete all of the reps in a set easily and with good form. For more information on how to find the best weight for each exercise, see the 10-Minute Life Changer on page 38.

(continued on page 38)

WHAT ABOUT CARDIO?

The Fit in 10 routines use metabolic circuit training to tone and sculpt the body while increasing your heart rate. While they aren't straight cardio, they provide some of the energy-boosting, heart-healthy benefits of cardio while helping you build metabolism-revving muscle mass. In fact, circuit training has been shown to offer comparable cardiovascular benefits to walking and jogging, according to a study published in the *Scandinavian Journal of Medicine & Science in Sports*.[6]

So if you're new to exercise or are just getting back to regular activity, follow the 60-day toning plan that begins on page 42, and do just one 10-minute routine each day. If you find that the 10-minute routines give you the energy to slip on your sneaks and get out there for a walk or a jog, go for it. You'll speed your metabolism further and score more of the amazing stress-reducing and mind-body benefits a little extra sweat can provide.

If you already walk, run, or do another form of cardiovascular activity that you enjoy, keep it up. Adding the Fit in 10 routines to your current regimen is going to help you break through weight loss plateaus and tone the zones that you've been struggling with, including the belly, butt, and upper arms.

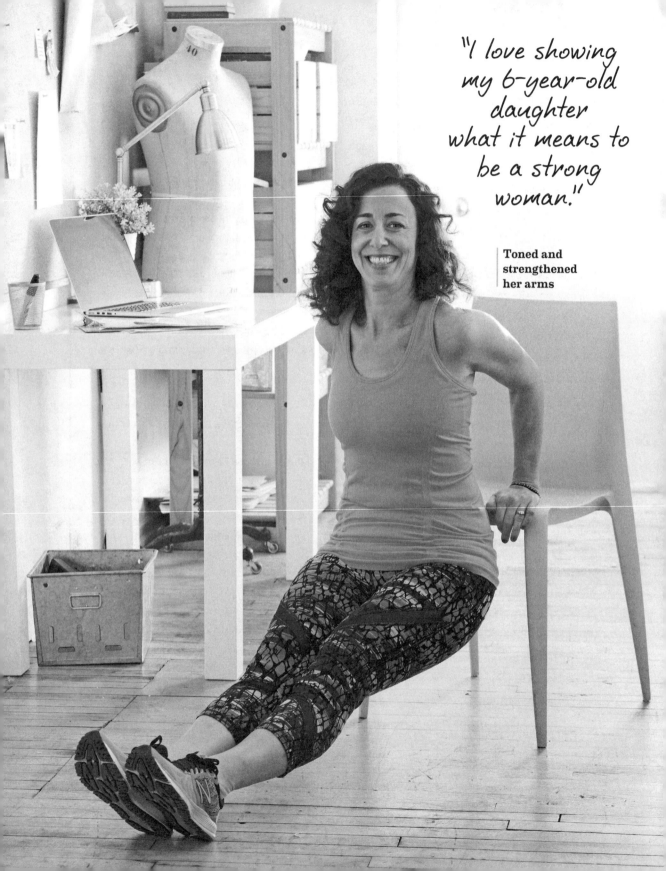

"I love showing my 6-year-old daughter what it means to be a strong woman."

Toned and strengthened her arms

Ali McDowell

AGE:	**46**
POUNDS LOST:	**10**
INCHES LOST:	**15.75**

Ali McDowell was doing one of the 10-minute routines in her living room when she noticed her 6-year-old daughter, Ruby, watching her intently from the couch. When Ali finished, she turned around and asked her daughter, "Why do you think Mommy exercises?" Ruby thought for a moment, then said: "To be a strong woman."

Her answer made the 46-year-old mom smile "One of my biggest motivators for doing this program was to show my daughter that eating right and exercising isn't just about being thin or pretty," says Ali, who works part-time for a nonprofit organization that educates children about food and nutrition. "As an older mom of a young child, I want to be healthy and strong for her for as long as possible."

Making that goal a reality became a lot easier when Ali discovered the power of Fit in 10. Like many women, she'd always struggled with her weight. "I have a memory of myself standing on a scale in my parents' bathroom when I was just 13 years old and being 150 pounds," Ali recalls. By the time she hit her thirties, her weight had crept past 180 pounds. She joined Weight Watchers and, even though she didn't enjoy it, started counting points and calories. While she lost about 20 pounds and kept it off over the next decade, managing her weight felt like constant battle. She'd go up a few pounds, lose it, then regain. Eight years ago, she went gluten-free in an effort to control her psoriasis. "It helped my skin, and a side benefit was that not eating bread or pasta made it easier for me to maintain my weight," says Ali. But even then, she still couldn't shake the last 10 pounds that had settled around her midsection.

Everything changed when Ali cleaned up her diet and started squeezing in the 10-minute sculpting routines. "In the past, I always knew what I was supposed to do when it came to healthy eating and exercise, but it was really tough to stick with anything because I'm a foodie with a really crazy schedule," she says.

The food plan appealed to Ali for multiple reasons. First, she loved that the recipes relied on fresh, whole foods. "They're really yummy and easy to put together. I couldn't believe that I could eat homemade food this delicious and still lose weight," she says. Second, it made her look at the labels of foods she always thought of as healthy more closely. "I was shocked to realize that many of the foods I kept in my pantry—like the sunflower seed butter I used to eat for breakfast every morning—were loaded with sugar," she says.

After 60 days, Ali couldn't believe the transformation. Not only had she dropped nearly 9 pounds, she could see a real difference in her body. "Overall, everything is tighter and more toned," she says. "I have more definition in my arms, my thighs look slimmer, and my abs are much stronger." Now, Ali is down a total of 10 pounds and isn't planning on stopping Fit in 10 anytime soon. "It's part of my lifestyle," she says.

Why Ali Loves Fit in 10

YOU CAN DO IT AT HOME. "My daughter hates the gym's day care, so it's really nice for both of us. I love spending more time with my family."

◀ BEFORE

A STURDY CHAIR. Many of the Fit in 10 moves are intended to challenge and develop your balance. Placing your hand on the back of a chair for a little extra support is a great way to build your strength and balance safely, especially when you're just starting out. Some of the upper body exercises can also be performed seated if you can't stand or you have difficulty standing. We'll also use the chair from time to time for some awesome sculpting exercises, like chair dips and hip lifts.

AN EXERCISE OR YOGA MAT. When it's time to hit the floor for ab work, a little extra cushion can go a long way. If you don't have a mat, don't sweat it; a carpeted surface will do just fine.

IO-MINUTE LIFE CHANGER
Find the Right Weight

In order to change your body, you have to challenge your body—and that's especially true when it comes to building lean, calorie-crushing muscle mass. "If you want to increase your strength or rebuild the muscle you've lost during the aging process, you probably need to pick up heavier weights," says strength-training expert Wayne Westcott, PhD. In addition to making the mistake of lifting too light, many women also tend to use the same set of dumbbells for every exercise. "Look at your thighs, then look at your arms," says Dr. Westcott. "Your leg muscles are much larger, and they need more weight than your biceps in order to be adequately challenged."

So how much should you lift for each exercise? "Determine the heaviest weight with which you can perform IO biceps curls with perfect form and control," says Dr. Westcott. Once you figure out the ideal weight, you can quickly factor how much you should use for other exercises using the chart below. "Everyone is different, but these numbers are calculated based on the average 50-year-old woman," says Dr. Westcott.

Try It! Sit tall on the edge of a sturdy chair, holding a dumbbell in each hand. If you haven't been strength training, start with 5-pound dumbbells. If you've been strength training, start with IO-pound dumbbells. Keeping your abs engaged and shoulders rolled down and back, start performing biceps curls by hinging the elbow and bringing the weights toward your shoulders. If you can do more than IO reps with perfect form, you need to increase the weight. If you can't reach IO without starting to strain or compromising on your form, you need to reduce the weight. Now that you know the best weight for your biceps curl, take a look at the chart in the sidebar on the opposite page.

How to Modify the Plan for Your Fitness Level

The Fit in 10 routines were carefully designed to maximize results while minimizing pain, discomfort, and risk of injury. However, every body is unique and it's important to listen to what yours is telling you. If you need to back off, back off. While there may be a few exercises that you might never perform due to a preexisting injury or condition, as you become stronger, you should find that many of the moves that originally seemed impossible are suddenly doable. Here are a few simple ways to achieve the results you want while being kind to your body.

IF YOUR KNEES BOTHER YOU . . . Take it slow, but try to keep moving. While it may

The Best Weight for Every Exercise

Upper Body Exercises			
EXERCISE	IF YOU CAN CURL 5 LB	IF YOU CAN CURL 8 LB	IF YOU CAN CURL 10 LB
TRICEPS KICKBACK (SAME)	5 lb	8 lb	10 lb
OVERHEAD TRICEPS EXTENSION (SAME TO 25% HIGHER)	5 to 6.25 lb	8 to 10 lb	10 to 12 lb
BENCH PRESS (25% TO 50% HIGHER)	6.25 to 7.5 lb	10 to 12 lb	12 to 15 lb
BENT-OVER ROW (25% TO 50% HIGHER)	6.25 to 7.5 lb	10 to 12 lb	12 to 15 lb
SHOULDER PRESS (SAME TO 25% HIGHER)	5 to 6.25 lb	8 to 10 lb	10 to 12 lb
SHOULDER SHRUG (25% TO 50% HIGHER)	6.25 to 7.5 lb	10 to 12 lb	12 to 15 lb
Lower Body Exercises			
EXERCISE	IF YOU CAN CURL 5 LB	IF YOU CAN CURL 8 LB	IF YOU CAN CURL 10 LB
SQUAT (50% TO 100% HIGHER)	7.5 to 10 lb	12 to 16 lb	15 to 20 lb
LUNGE (SAME TO 25% HIGHER)	5 to 6.25 lb	8 to 10 lb	10 to 12 lb
HEEL RAISE (50% TO 100% HIGHER)	7.5 to 10 lb	12 to 16 lb	15 to 20 lb

sound counterintuitive, research shows that regular exercise can greatly reduce chronic knee pain in a large majority of sufferers. In fact, a recent study published in *BMJ* found that when women and men with chronic knee pain performed simple, at-home exercises that strengthened the supportive muscles around the knee two or three times a week for 12 weeks, the reduction in pain was so significant that more than half of the study participants felt they no longer needed knee surgery.[7] Many of these same exercises, like squats and lunges, are used in the Fit in 10 routines. If you find these moves too challenging at first, modify them by not bending your knees as deeply. You can also place your hands on the back of a chair for balance. If that's too difficult, you can sub in the step-up exercise described in the box below. It will work the muscles in your butt and thighs without requiring you to hinge at the hips or bend so deeply into the knees.

TRY IT!

Stand tall with your abs engaged in front of a stair, exercise step, or plyo box (the higher the step, the more challenging the exercise). Place your right foot on the step, then your left foot. Reverse the movement. Continue stepping up and down for 30 seconds. Repeat the movement for another 30 seconds, this time leading with your left foot.

IF YOU CAN'T PUT WEIGHT ON YOUR HANDS . . . Rethink common floor exercises. Planks and pushups are two of the most effective exercises for strengthening and sculpting the upper body and core, but they can be uncomfortable for anyone with achy wrists or hands. You can still enjoy their benefits, however, simply by doing these moves with your hands on an elevated surface. So if you find knee pushups or planks incredibly challenging, take them to the wall (see pages 71 and 86 for an example). When wall exercises become too easy, place your hands on the seat of a sturdy chair. The closer your body gets to the floor, the more weight you'll place on your hands and wrists. Eventually, as you increase your strength and flexibility, you may be able to bring planks and pushups back down to the floor. In the meantime, you'll tone a killer core and upper body.

IF YOU CAN'T GET DOWN ON THE FLOOR . . . Stay positive! Many of the Fit in 10 moves, like band walks and biceps curls, naturally take place seated or standing. Additionally, exercises that are normally done on the floor, like bicycle crunches, can often be modified to a seated or standing variation that offers similar benefits. If there's a move that doesn't have a viable modification for you, simply walk in place or step side to side. Just keeping your heart rate up for 10 minutes is going to have a big effect on your health, energy, and body.

Your Fit in 10 Training Plan

It's time to get toned in 10. Following this training plan will help you get stronger and slimmer in just 60 days by showing you how to mix and match the Fit in 10 routines for weight loss and all-over toning. It's the exact program that our test panelists used to drop up to 18 pounds and 24 combined inches from their belly, waist, hips, thighs, and upper arms in 8 weeks.

The Fit in 10 training plan is broken up into six 10-day cycles that become progressively more challenging so you never get bored and you continue to see results. Many of our test panelists loved that they could tackle the plan 10 days at a time. "When I thought about doing each 10-day cycle separately, it felt a lot more doable than when I thought of committing to the training plan for a full 60 days," says Eileen Clark. "I just told myself, start with 10 days, and see how you feel. By cycle 2, I knew I would finish. I was already getting hooked on how good it felt to strengthen and move my body."

Each day, you'll complete one of the 10-minute routines that start on page 47. (Starting in cycle 3, you'll have the option to add a second routine. These are optional; only do them if you have the energy and time for an extra challenge!) While sticking with the daily plan will speed your results while helping you create a lifelong habit of regular weight training, there may be days when you miss a workout or want a day off. When that happens, you can stack two workouts on the following day to make up the time. Just do your best to get right back to the daily schedule.

10-MINUTE LIFE CHANGER
Commit to a Morning Workout

If your day is a nonstop marathon from start to finish, setting your alarm 10 minutes earlier so you can do your Fit in 10 routine before the rush begins could greatly increase your chances of success. Research shows that morning exercisers are much more likely to follow through with their intention to work out than those who plan to do so in the evening.[8] The scientific theory: Willpower is a limited, renewable resource. You start the day with a certain amount in the bank, and each time you make a decision, resist a temptation, or check your emotions, you make a withdrawal from the willpower bank. By the time the evening hits and you're faced with the decision to work out or fall onto the couch, there's often little brainpower left to make the right decision. So, if you are struggling with consistency, make it a goal to squeeze in your sculpting before you hop into the shower. I promise that you'll start the day feeling like superwoman.

Your 60-Day Fit in 10 Training Plan

Your transformation starts here. Do the workout that's listed each day,
and don't forget to journal your progress.

Cycle 1	Lean and Lovely Legs	Back to Strong	Deep Core	Happy Hipster
	1	**2**	**3**	**4**
Cycle 2	Tummy Love	Ultimate Booty Lifter	Dare to Bare Arms	Sizzle and Sculpt
	11	**12**	**13**	**14**
Cycle 3	Flat and Firm Abs	Ultimate Booty Lifter	Totally Toned Triceps	Torch to Tone
	21	**22**	**23**	**24**
Cycle 4	Lean and Lovely Legs	Totally Toned Triceps	Sizzle and Sculpt	Back to Strong / Deep Core*
	31	**32**	**33**	**34**
Cycle 5	Meta Blast / Deep Core*	Lean and Lovely Legs	Dare to Bare Arms / Tummy Love*	Torch to Tone
	41	**42**	**43**	**44**
Cycle 6	Ultimate Booty Lifter / Tummy Love*	Sizzle and Sculpt	Lean and Lovely Legs / Back to Strong*	Dare to Bare Arms
	51	**52**	**53**	**54**

Tone Zone | Lower Body

Happy Hipster (page 50)
Ultimate Booty Lifter (page 56)
Lean and Lovely Legs (page 62)

Tone Zone | Upper Body

Dare to Bare Arms (page 70)
Totally Toned Triceps (page 76)
Back to Strong (page 82)

Dare to Bare Arms	Flat and Firm Abs	Ultimate Booty Lifter	Totally Toned Triceps	Lean and Lovely Legs	Meta Blast
5	**6**	**7**	**8**	**9**	**10**
Deep Core	Happy Hipster	Back to Strong	Flat and Firm Abs	Meta Blast	Lean and Lovely Legs
15	**16**	**17**	**18**	**19**	**20**
Back to Strong	Sizzle and Sculpt	Dare to Bare Arms / Deep Core*	Happy Hipster	Tummy Love	Meta Blast
25	**26**	**27**	**28**	**29**	**30**
Ultimate Booty Lifter	Meta Blast	Dare to Bare Arms	Happy Hipster	Torch to Tone / Tummy Love*	Flat and Firm Abs
35	**36**	**37**	**38**	**39**	**40**
Totally Toned Triceps / Flat and Firm Abs*	Ultimate Booty Lifter	Sizzle and Sculpt	Lean and Lovely Legs / Back to Strong*	Flat and Firm Abs	Meta Blast
45	**46**	**47**	**48**	**49**	**50**
Meta Blast / Deep Core*	Happy Hipster	Torch to Tone	Ultimate Booty Lifter / Totally Toned Triceps*	Flat and Firm Abs / Lean and Lovely Legs*	Sizzle and Sculpt
55	**56**	**57**	**58**	**59**	**60**

Tone Zone | Belly

Flat and Firm Abs (page 90)
Deep Core (page 96)
Tummy Love (page 102)

Tone Zone | Total Body

Sizzle and Sculpt (page 110)
Meta Blast (page 116)
Torch to Tone (page 122)

* = Optional second workout

10-MINUTE LIFE CHANGER
Take a Stretch Break

When you're crunched for time, stretching is often the first part of your workout routine that gets discarded. Then, after months of ignoring your hamstrings, you bend over to tie your shoes and your feet suddenly seem miles away. The good news: You can loosen up, increase your flexibility, and maximize your mobility by building up to 10 minutes of stretching a few times a week. Not only will it feel great—and help you move through life with more ease—you'll be less likely to need that ibuprofen. When women and men with chronic low back pain stretched at home at least three times a week, they reported a significant decrease in pain levels in just 12 weeks, according to a study published in the *Archives of Internal Medicine*.[9] Plus, it's a major stress reliever. "I always feel so much better after taking a few minutes to stretch my muscles," says 54-year-old test panelist Wendy Marcus. "Sometimes I'll stretch right after my Fit in 10 routines, and sometimes I'll stretch after a long period of inactivity. No matter when I do it, I feel more calm and refreshed when I'm done." Here are a few simple stretches to get you started.

CHEST OPENER Stand with your arms hanging in front of your thighs, holding a belt or strap with your hands slightly more than shoulder-width apart. Keeping your arms straight, raise your arms in an arc overhead and back behind you. Pause, then slowly reverse the movement to the starting position. Continue for 30 seconds.

CALF STRETCH Stand about 2 feet from a wall, facing it in a staggered stance, one foot in front of the other. Keeping your back heel down, place your hands on the wall and lean against it. Hold for 30 seconds, then switch legs and repeat. Stretch each leg twice.

HAMSTRING STRETCH Lie on your back with your knees bent and your feet flat on the floor, holding one end of a belt or strap in each hand. Draw one knee in toward your chest and place the middle of the strap around the arch of your foot. Extend your leg toward the ceiling, holding for 30 seconds. Repeat with the other leg. Stretch each leg twice.

HIP FLEXOR STRETCH Start by kneeling on the floor. Place your right foot in front of you, then slowly press your hips forward until you feel a stretch in front of your left thigh. Hold for 30 seconds. Repeat with the other leg. Stretch each leg twice.

QUAD STRETCH Stand tall with one hand on the back of a sturdy chair for support. Bend one knee and grab the top of your foot with your hand, pulling it toward your body and pushing your hips forward until you feel a stretch in the front of the thigh. Hold for 30 seconds. Repeat with the other leg. Stretch each leg twice.

Sarah M.

AGE:	**33**
POUNDS LOST:	**18**
INCHES LOST:	**23.75**

When Sarah crossed the finish line of a half marathon this past spring, she should have been proud. When the 33-year-old accounting and HR consultant realized she finished the 13.1-mile race 45 minutes behind her friends, however, her excitement diminished. "I hated being the slowest one."

Sarah knew what was slowing her down: Over the past 2 years, despite training for a few races, she'd struggled to maintain her weight, and it had slowly crept up to 220 pounds. Single life in New York City–late nights out with friends and the high-calorie fast food she tended to grab on the go when she didn't feel like cooking–had caught up with her.

It was frustrating, but Sarah wasn't surprised. Her struggle with the scale started in high school. "Ever since then, I've either been on a diet or feeling like I should go on a diet," she recalls. "I've had a few really successful periods of getting fit, but then there is always some trigger–or maybe just a loosening of standards–and little by little I would undo all the hard work."

When Sarah heard about the *Fit in 10: Slim & Strong–for Life!* program on *Prevention*'s Facebook page, the simplicity of the plan appealed to her. "I really liked that it was manageable," she says.

Still, Sarah wasn't so sure the 10-minute workouts would challenge her. In the past, she had an all-or-nothing mentality when it came to exercise.

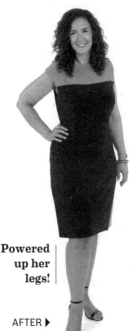

Powered up her legs!

AFTER ▶

"I thought anything less than an hour wasn't a 'real' workout," she says. Once she started following the Fit in 10 plan, she was happily surprised. "I thought they were going to be too short to have an impact, but they were really challenging," she says. "The only easy part about them was getting them done. A few times, I even did my workout in my pajamas before climbing into bed."

Following the Fit in 10 meal plan gave Sarah a sense of calm and control. "The rules made it easy to make the right decisions without making me feel super restricted," she says.

Within a few weeks of starting the Fit in 10 plan, Sarah noticed a major difference. She felt more cheerful, less stressed, and her lower body looked tighter. Seven weeks in, though, was when she realized that Fit in 10 was changing more than just her body. "I went for a run, and–thanks to weighing less and having stronger legs–I felt so fast and light. It was amazing."

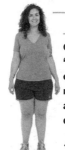

Why Sarah Loves Fit in 10

ONE FIT IN 10 MEAL CAN FEED YOU ALL WEEK: "The poached salmon (page 225) was one of my go-to dinners. It was so simple to make and really delicious. I'd make extra and eat it cold on salads or sandwiches on days when I didn't have time to cook."

◀ BEFORE

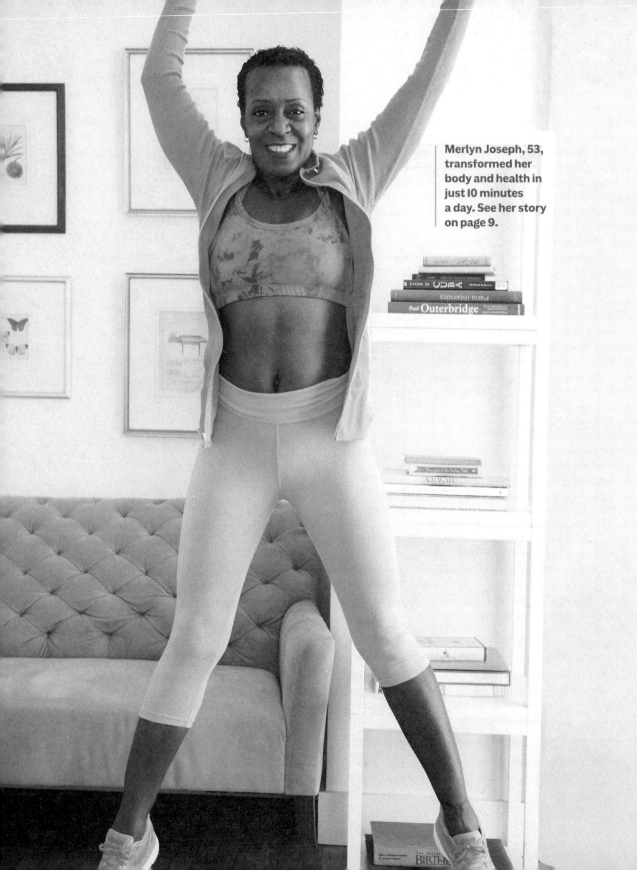

Merlyn Joseph, 53, transformed her body and health in just 10 minutes a day. See her story on page 9.

5

The 10-Minute Workouts

You already know that regular exercise is one of the best ways to transform your health and body. Unfortunately, it's not always easy—or even possible—to find the time and motivation to commit to 30 to 60 minutes each day. That's why I worked with my friend and trainer Larysa DiDio (who demonstrates the moves in the following pages) to design these fast and fun routines that target common trouble spots in just 10 minutes a day. In addition to firming and sculpting your body in the time it takes to check your email, they'll also increase your strength and stamina and kick your metabolism into overdrive. I've divided them into Tone Zones so you can quickly find the best routine for your goals or for your mood and energy levels that day. Each zone hits a specific area—upper body, lower body, belly, and total body—while increasing calorie burn. Many of the routines also include simple moves that quickly build your mobility and balance so you can move through your day with power and fewer aches and pains.

"Even with all of my craziness, I'm able fit them into my day," says Christine Szpynda. "Within days of being on the program, I started to see changes in strength, energy, and body." Now, it's your turn. Turn the page to discover how to get stronger and slimmer and tone every zone in just 10 minutes a day.

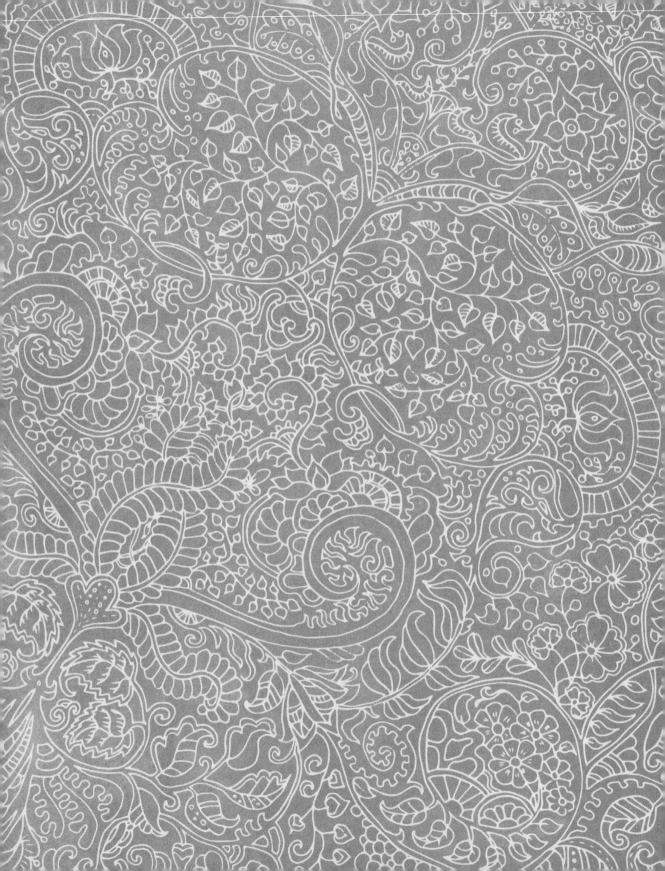

LOWER BODY

These 10-minute routines will help you sculpt a stronger, shapelier lower body. Within a few weeks, you'll notice leaner, sleeker legs that will power you through your day. Bonus: You'll look amazing in jeans and dresses, too. "I loved doing a different workout each day and that 10 minutes could really kick my butt," says Ali McDowell, 46, who lost 10 pounds and 15.75 inches in 60 days.

HAPPY HIPSTER

Shape and firm your beautiful hips and thighs with these effective moves that require nothing more than a resistance band loop and a chair. The bands are gentle and easy to use, but don't be surprised when your lower body starts to shake; they add an extra challenge by keeping tension on the muscles throughout the full motion of each rep.

How to do it: Choose a resistance band strength that works best for your body. Do each exercise for 40 seconds. Rest for 20 seconds between exercises as you transition to the next move. Do the circuit twice.

① Band Squat

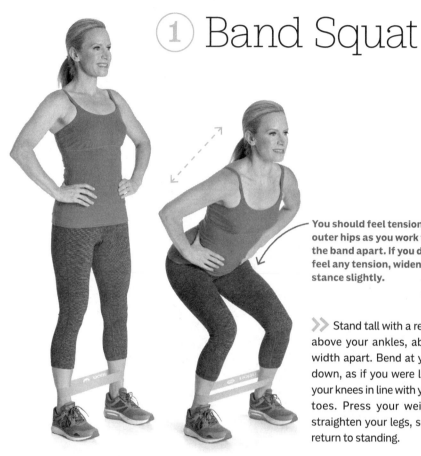

You should feel tension in the outer hips as you work to keep the band apart. If you don't feel any tension, widen your stance slightly.

›› Stand tall with a resistance band loop slightly above your ankles, abs engaged, and feet hip-width apart. Bend at your hips and sit back and down, as if you were lowering into a chair. Keep your knees in line with your ankles and behind your toes. Press your weight into your heels and straighten your legs, squeezing your butt as you return to standing.

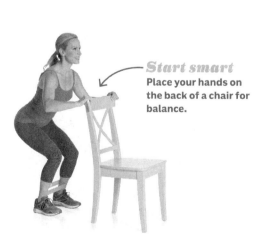

Start smart
Place your hands on the back of a chair for balance.

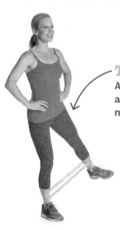

Tone faster
As you return to standing, add a lateral leg lift. Alternate legs with each rep.

② Split Squat 'n' Squeeze

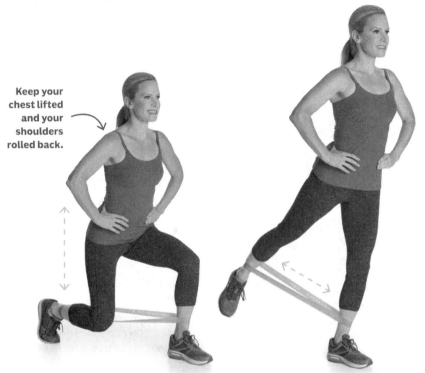

Keep your chest lifted and your shoulders rolled back.

>> Stand tall with a resistance band loop slightly above your ankles, abs engaged, and feet hip-width apart. Step your right leg behind you, balancing on the ball of your right foot. This is your starting position. Now bend both of your knees, back knee lowering toward the floor, coming into a split squat. As you prepare to stand back up, press your weight into your left heel and straighten your leg as you lift your right leg behind you. Lower your right foot to the floor to return to your starting position. Continue for 20 seconds; repeat on the opposite side for another 20 seconds.

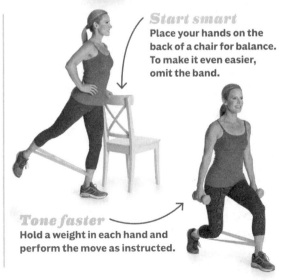

Start smart
Place your hands on the back of a chair for balance. To make it even easier, omit the band.

Tone faster
Hold a weight in each hand and perform the move as instructed.

③ Thigh Sweep

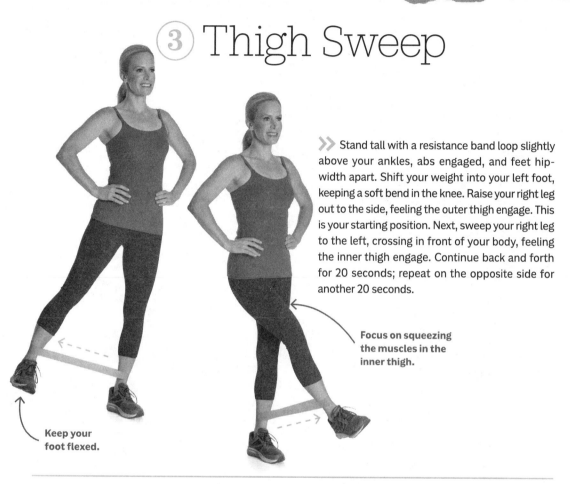

>> Stand tall with a resistance band loop slightly above your ankles, abs engaged, and feet hip-width apart. Shift your weight into your left foot, keeping a soft bend in the knee. Raise your right leg out to the side, feeling the outer thigh engage. This is your starting position. Next, sweep your right leg to the left, crossing in front of your body, feeling the inner thigh engage. Continue back and forth for 20 seconds; repeat on the opposite side for another 20 seconds.

Focus on squeezing the muscles in the inner thigh.

Keep your foot flexed.

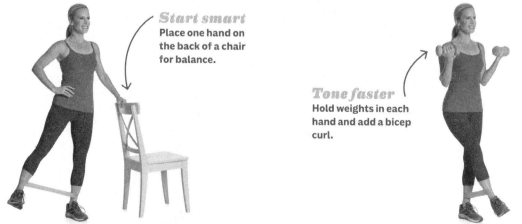

Start smart
Place one hand on the back of a chair for balance.

Tone faster
Hold weights in each hand and add a bicep curl.

④ Standing Leg Raise

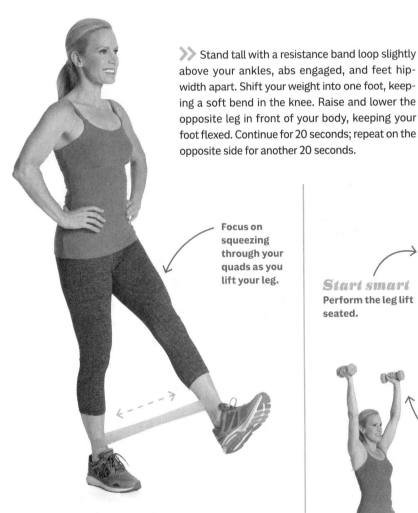

>> Stand tall with a resistance band loop slightly above your ankles, abs engaged, and feet hip-width apart. Shift your weight into one foot, keeping a soft bend in the knee. Raise and lower the opposite leg in front of your body, keeping your foot flexed. Continue for 20 seconds; repeat on the opposite side for another 20 seconds.

Focus on squeezing through your quads as you lift your leg.

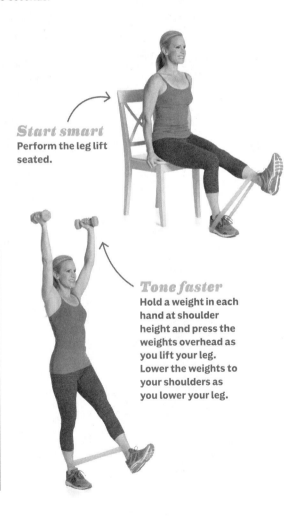

Start smart
Perform the leg lift seated.

Tone faster
Hold a weight in each hand at shoulder height and press the weights overhead as you lift your leg. Lower the weights to your shoulders as you lower your leg.

⑤ Half-Star Hop

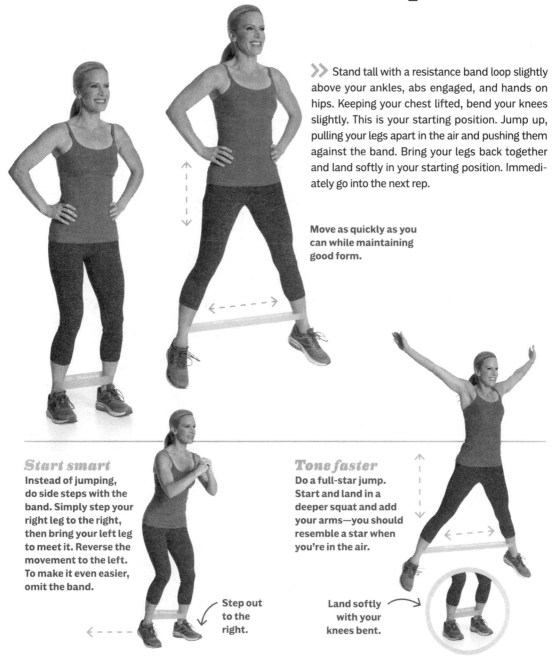

≫ Stand tall with a resistance band loop slightly above your ankles, abs engaged, and hands on hips. Keeping your chest lifted, bend your knees slightly. This is your starting position. Jump up, pulling your legs apart in the air and pushing them against the band. Bring your legs back together and land softly in your starting position. Immediately go into the next rep.

Move as quickly as you can while maintaining good form.

Start smart
Instead of jumping, do side steps with the band. Simply step your right leg to the right, then bring your left leg to meet it. Reverse the movement to the left. To make it even easier, omit the band.

Step out to the right.

Tone faster
Do a full-star jump. Start and land in a deeper squat and add your arms—you should resemble a star when you're in the air.

Land softly with your knees bent.

ULTIMATE BOOTY LIFTER

Tone and tighten your backside with this kick-butt routine. It hits the glutes from every angle to help you build a stronger and more lifted seat in just 10 minutes. All you need is a chair; add a resistance band loop and hand weights for an extra challenge.

How to do it: Do 2 rounds of Circuit 1, then do 2 rounds of Circuit 2. Perform each exercise for 40 seconds, and rest for 20 seconds as you transition to the next move.

① Curtsy Lunge to Lateral Leg Lift

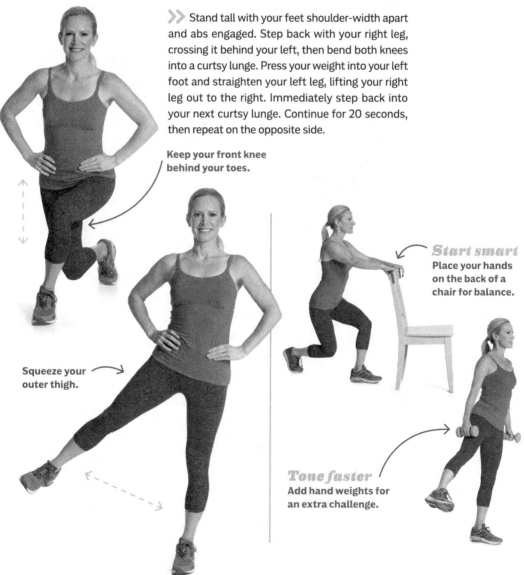

>> Stand tall with your feet shoulder-width apart and abs engaged. Step back with your right leg, crossing it behind your left, then bend both knees into a curtsy lunge. Press your weight into your left foot and straighten your left leg, lifting your right leg out to the right. Immediately step back into your next curtsy lunge. Continue for 20 seconds, then repeat on the opposite side.

Keep your front knee behind your toes.

Squeeze your outer thigh.

Start smart
Place your hands on the back of a chair for balance.

Tone faster
Add hand weights for an extra challenge.

② Step-Back Lunge with a Squeeze

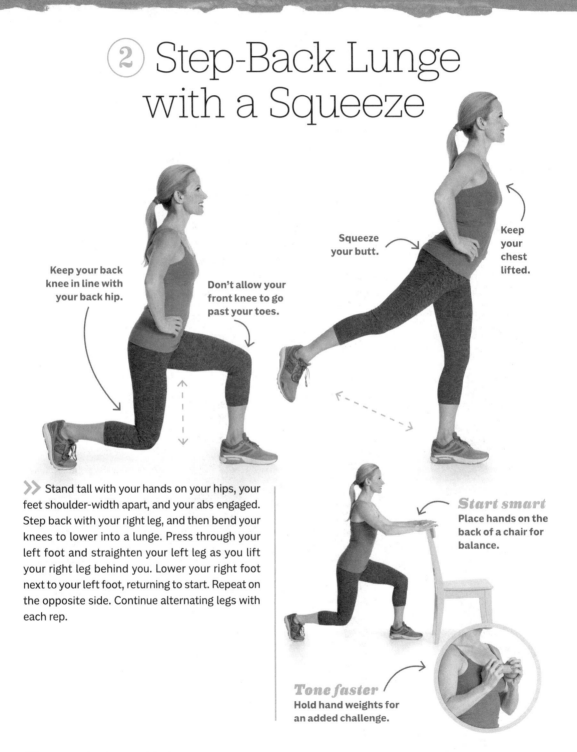

Keep your back knee in line with your back hip.

Don't allow your front knee to go past your toes.

Squeeze your butt.

Keep your chest lifted.

Start smart
Place hands on the back of a chair for balance.

Tone faster
Hold hand weights for an added challenge.

» Stand tall with your hands on your hips, your feet shoulder-width apart, and your abs engaged. Step back with your right leg, and then bend your knees to lower into a lunge. Press through your left foot and straighten your left leg as you lift your right leg behind you. Lower your right foot next to your left foot, returning to start. Repeat on the opposite side. Continue alternating legs with each rep.

③ Single-Leg Chair Squat

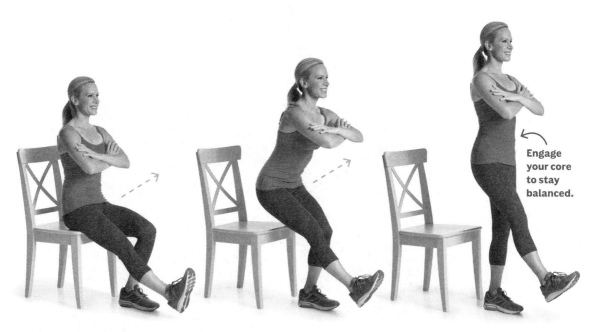

Engage
your core
to stay
balanced.

>> Sit tall on the edge of a chair with your arms crossed, your left foot on the floor, and your right leg extended and elevated a few inches off the floor. Engage your abs and lean your torso forward slightly, then firmly press your weight into your left foot and straighten your left leg to a standing position. Slowly press your hips back and lower your butt back to the chair. Continue for 20 seconds; repeat on the opposite side for another 20 seconds.

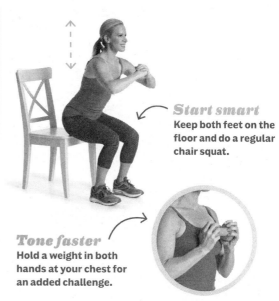

Start smart
Keep both feet on the
floor and do a regular
chair squat.

Tone faster
Hold a weight in both
hands at your chest for
an added challenge.

CIRCUIT 2: FLOOR

④ Marching Bridge

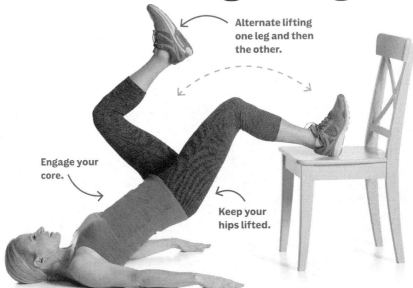

Alternate lifting one leg and then the other.

Engage your core.

Keep your hips lifted.

>> Lie on your back with your heels on the edge of a chair seat, knees bent at 90 degrees. Press your heels into the chair seat and lift your hips until your body forms a straight line. This is your starting position. Hold here, and begin marching your legs. Lift one leg, lower it back to the seat, then lift the other. Continue alternating legs for the duration of the set.

Start smart
Omit the marches. Simply hold the bridge, taking rests when needed.

Tone faster
Keep your legs straight and perform the move as directed.

⑤ Forearm Plank with Hip Hyperextension

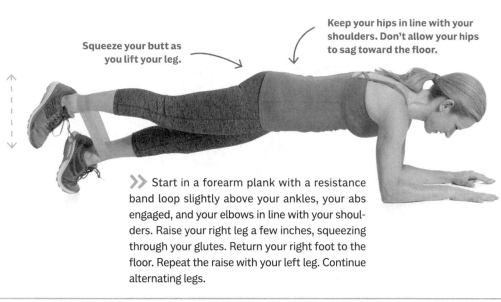

Squeeze your butt as you lift your leg.

Keep your hips in line with your shoulders. Don't allow your hips to sag toward the floor.

» Start in a forearm plank with a resistance band loop slightly above your ankles, your abs engaged, and your elbows in line with your shoulders. Raise your right leg a few inches, squeezing through your glutes. Return your right foot to the floor. Repeat the raise with your left leg. Continue alternating legs.

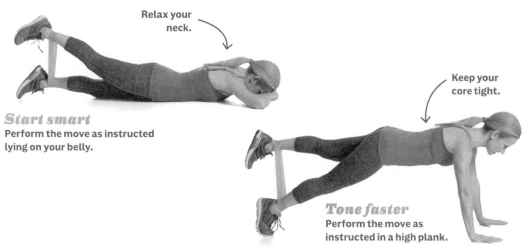

Relax your neck.

Keep your core tight.

Start smart
Perform the move as instructed lying on your belly.

Tone faster
Perform the move as instructed in a high plank.

LEAN AND LOVELY LEGS

This 10-minute routine combines ridiculously effective lower body moves with resistance band loops and hand weights to totally transform your legs. In just five simple moves, you'll firm and strengthen the glutes, calves, and inner and outer thighs.

How to do it: Do Circuit I twice, and do Circuit 2 twice. Perform each exercise for 40 seconds, and rest for 20 seconds as you transition to the next move.

① Tiptoe Squat

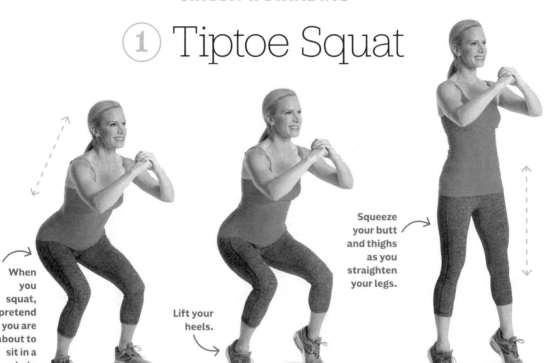

When you squat, pretend you are about to sit in a chair.

Lift your heels.

Squeeze your butt and thighs as you straighten your legs.

>> Stand tall with your feet hip-width apart, abs engaged, and chest lifted. Bend at your hips and sit back and down into a squat. Lift your heels, then press through the balls of your feet and straighten legs to return to standing. Lower heels and move into the next squat.

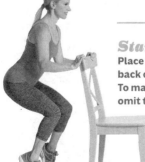

Start smart
Place your hands on the back of a chair for balance. To make it even easier, omit the heel raise.

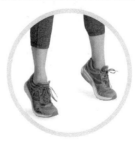

Tone faster
Don't lower your heels back to the ground; stay on your tiptoes the entire time.

② Lunge and Lift

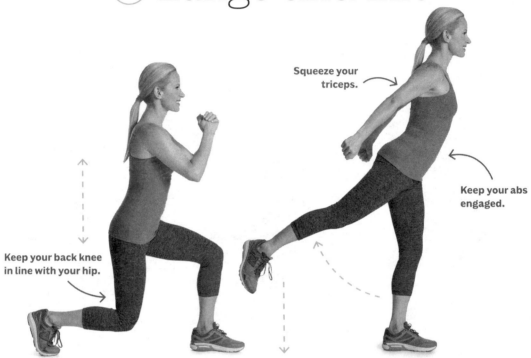

Squeeze your triceps.

Keep your abs engaged.

Keep your back knee in line with your hip.

>> Stand tall in a split stance with your right leg a few feet behind your left leg. Bend both of your knees to lower into a lunge. Hold here and pulse three times, raising and lowering your hips a few inches. Next, lean your torso slightly forward and balance on your left leg as you lift your right leg and arms behind you, squeezing the glutes and triceps. Return your right foot to the floor and immediately lower into another lunge. Continue with the movement for 20 seconds, then repeat on the opposite side for another 20 seconds.

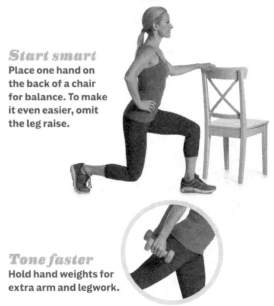

Start smart
Place one hand on the back of a chair for balance. To make it even easier, omit the leg raise.

Tone faster
Hold hand weights for extra arm and legwork.

③ Sumo Squat

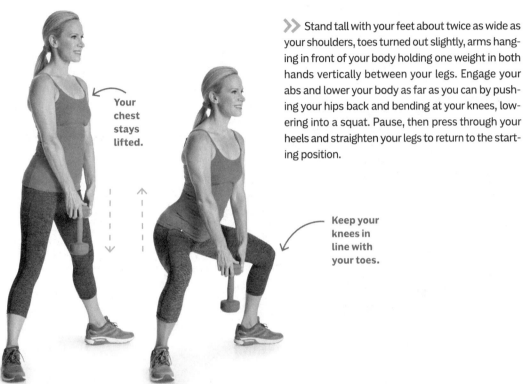

Your chest stays lifted.

>> Stand tall with your feet about twice as wide as your shoulders, toes turned out slightly, arms hanging in front of your body holding one weight in both hands vertically between your legs. Engage your abs and lower your body as far as you can by pushing your hips back and bending at your knees, lowering into a squat. Pause, then press through your heels and straighten your legs to return to the starting position.

Keep your knees in line with your toes.

Start smart
Place your hands on the back of a chair for balance.

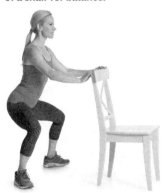

Tone faster
Do sumo squat jumps. Stand tall with your feet hip-width apart, abs engaged, and chest lifted. Jump your feet up and out, landing in a sumo squat. Jump your feet back to the starting position.

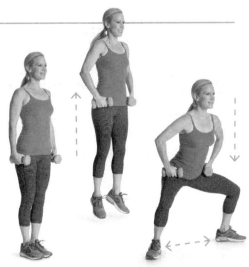

CIRCUIT 2: FLOOR

④ Thigh Slimmer

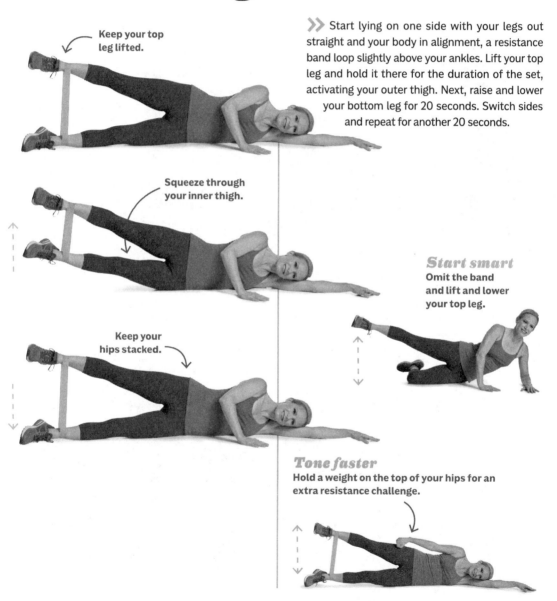

Keep your top leg lifted.

Squeeze through your inner thigh.

Keep your hips stacked.

>> Start lying on one side with your legs out straight and your body in alignment, a resistance band loop slightly above your ankles. Lift your top leg and hold it there for the duration of the set, activating your outer thigh. Next, raise and lower your bottom leg for 20 seconds. Switch sides and repeat for another 20 seconds.

Start smart
Omit the band and lift and lower your top leg.

Tone faster
Hold a weight on the top of your hips for an extra resistance challenge.

⑤ Seated Leg Raise

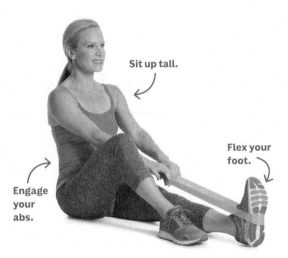

Sit up tall.

Engage your abs.

Flex your foot.

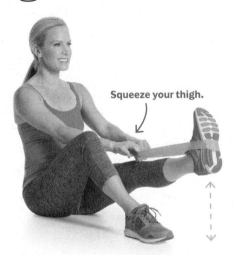

Squeeze your thigh.

>> Sit on the floor with your right knee bent and your right foot flat on the floor, your left leg extended in front of you. Place one end of the band around the bottom of your left foot and hold the other end with both hands. Raise and lower your left leg. Continue for 20 seconds and repeat on the opposite side for another 20 seconds.

Start smart
Place your hands on the floor and lean back slightly. Omit the band.

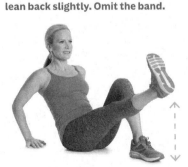

Tone faster
Place the resistance band loop around the ankle of the extended leg, and step on the other end of the band with your opposite foot. Raise and lower the extended leg.

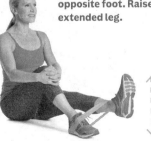

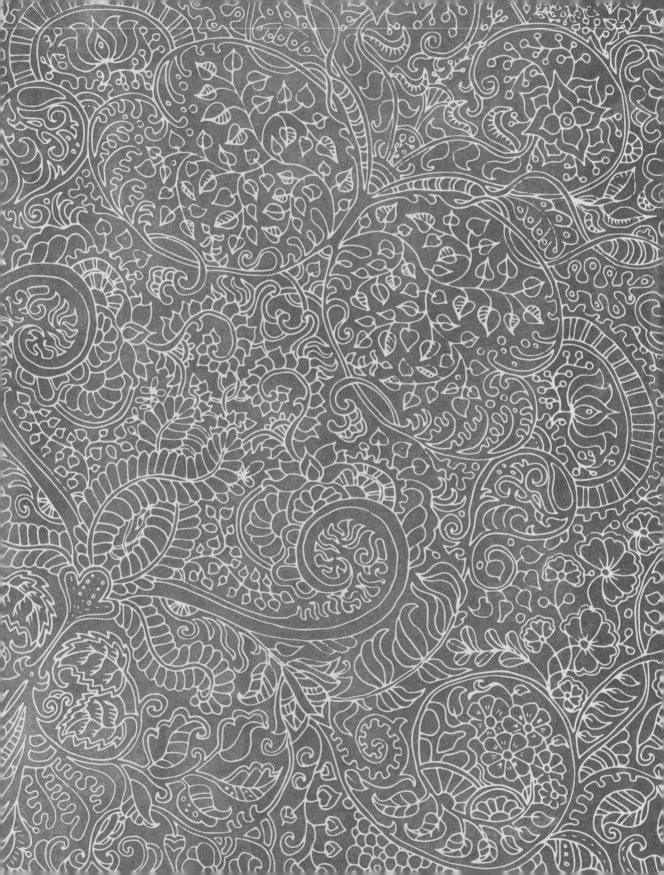

UPPER BODY

If you want strong, lean arms that look good in tank tops and are capable of carrying groceries, picking up kids, and hoisting heavy suitcases into the over-head bin, these 10-minute routines will help you get there. These do-anywhere moves beautifully sculpt your biceps, triceps, shoulders, and upper back while being gentle on your joints. "The routines really helped me take my upper body to the next level," says Linda Cohen, 45.

DARE TO BARE ARMS

Every inch of your upper body is challenged in this fast and fun 10-minute routine that incorporates key moves every woman needs for a strong upper body. You'll strengthen your chest, shoulders, biceps, and triceps in minutes. Grab your weights and a chair, and start toning!

How to do it: Perform each exercise for 20 seconds, and rest for 10 seconds as you transition to the next move. Do the circuit 4 times.

① Knee Pushup

>> Kneel on the floor with your hands directly beneath your shoulders and your legs bent so that your body is in a straight line from your head to your knees. Keep your elbows out to the sides and lower your chest to the floor. Hold for a second, and push back up.

Knees hurt? Use a mat or towel to cushion them.

Engage your abs to protect your lower back.

Lower your chest all the way to the floor.

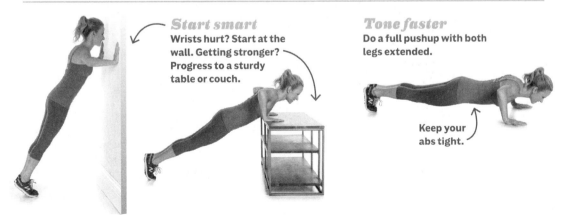

Start smart
Wrists hurt? Start at the wall. Getting stronger? Progress to a sturdy table or couch.

Tone faster
Do a full pushup with both legs extended.

Keep your abs tight.

② Hammer Curl to Shoulder Press

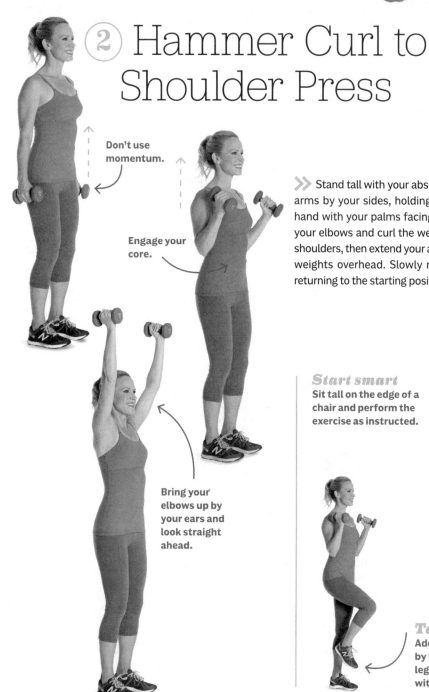

Don't use momentum.

Engage your core.

>> Stand tall with your abs engaged and your arms by your sides, holding a weight in each hand with your palms facing your body. Bend your elbows and curl the weights toward your shoulders, then extend your arms and press the weights overhead. Slowly reverse the move, returning to the starting position.

Bring your elbows up by your ears and look straight ahead.

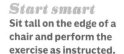

Start smart
Sit tall on the edge of a chair and perform the exercise as instructed.

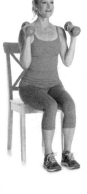

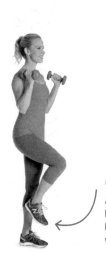

Tone faster
Add a core challenge by balancing on one leg; alternate legs with each set.

③ Pull-Press

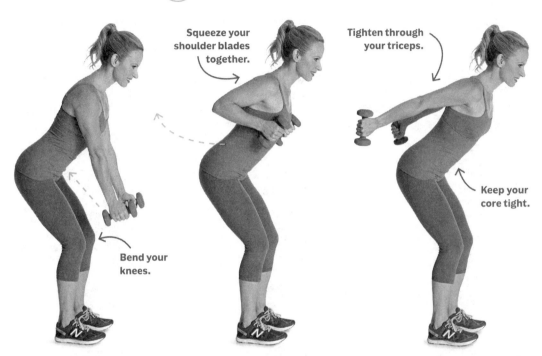

Squeeze your shoulder blades together.

Bend your knees.

Tighten through your triceps.

Keep your core tight.

>> Stand tall with your feet hip-width apart and your arms by your sides, holding one weight in each hand. Keeping your back flat and abs engaged, hinge forward at your hips, arms hanging toward the floor with palms facing each other. This is your starting position. Pull your elbows to your sides, then press the weights behind you. Slowly reverse the movement to the starting position.

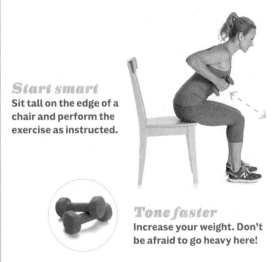

Start smart
Sit tall on the edge of a chair and perform the exercise as instructed.

Tone faster
Increase your weight. Don't be afraid to go heavy here!

④ Side Lateral Raise to Front Raise

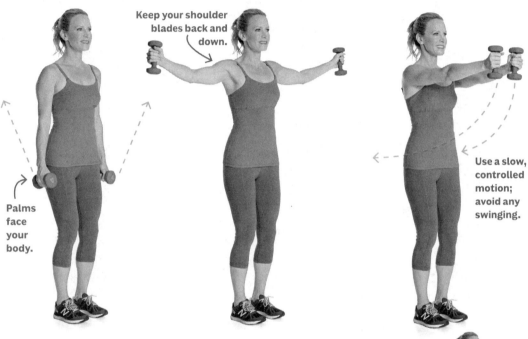

Keep your shoulder blades back and down.

Palms face your body.

Use a slow, controlled motion; avoid any swinging.

▶▶ Stand tall with your feet hip-width apart and your arms by your sides, holding one weight in each hand. Keeping your elbows slightly bent, raise the weights out to your sides to shoulder height. At the top of the exercise, move the weights out in front of you, keeping your arms extended. Lower the weights in front of your body and bring them back to your sides with a controlled motion. Slowly reverse the movement, raising the weights in front of you to shoulder height before moving the weights laterally to your sides. Lower the weights to the starting position. Continue alternating, first lifting the weights out to the sides and then out in front of you for the duration of the set.

Start smart
Sit tall on the edge of a chair and perform the exercise as instructed.

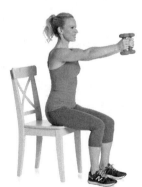

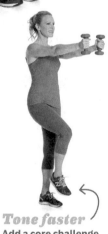

Tone faster
Add a core challenge by balancing on one leg; alternate legs with each set.

⑤ External Rotation to Chest Fly

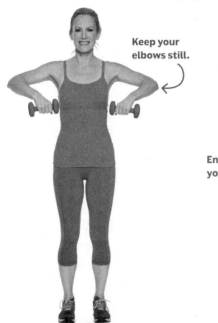

Keep your elbows still.

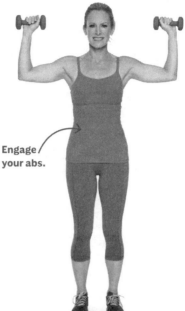

Engage your abs.

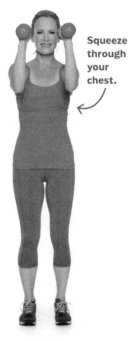

Squeeze through your chest.

>> Stand tall with your feet hip-width apart and your arms at shoulder height, elbows bent, holding one weight in each hand with palms facing down. Keeping your elbows still, rotate your shoulders to "goalpost arms," bringing your wrists over your elbows. Next, draw your elbows together in front of you, squeezing through your chest. Slowly reverse the movement back to start.

Start smart
Sit tall on the edge of a chair and perform the exercise as instructed.

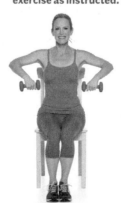

Tone faster
Increase your weight. Don't be afraid to go heavy here!

TOTALLY TONED TRICEPS

If the back of your upper arms could use some toning, this routine will help you do it in just 10 minutes. It combines resistance band work with light weights and body weight to firm and strengthen the triceps in the least amount of time.

How to do it: Perform each exercise for 20 seconds, and rest for 10 seconds as you transition to the next move. Do the circuit 4 times.

① Overhead Triceps Extension

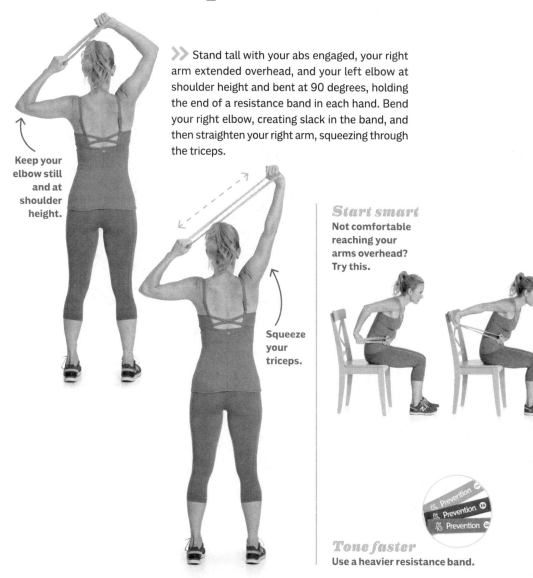

>> Stand tall with your abs engaged, your right arm extended overhead, and your left elbow at shoulder height and bent at 90 degrees, holding the end of a resistance band in each hand. Bend your right elbow, creating slack in the band, and then straighten your right arm, squeezing through the triceps.

Keep your elbow still and at shoulder height.

Squeeze your triceps.

Start smart
Not comfortable reaching your arms overhead? Try this.

Tone faster
Use a heavier resistance band.

② Triceps Push-Back

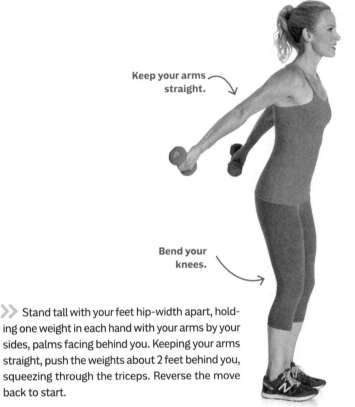

Keep your arms straight.

Bend your knees.

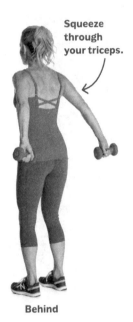

Squeeze through your triceps.

Behind

>> Stand tall with your feet hip-width apart, holding one weight in each hand with your arms by your sides, palms facing behind you. Keeping your arms straight, push the weights about 2 feet behind you, squeezing through the triceps. Reverse the move back to start.

Start smart
Perform the exercise seated. To make it easier, omit the weights.

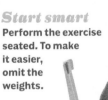
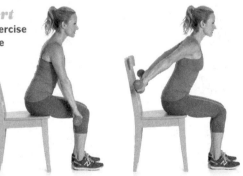

Tone faster
Use heavier weights.

③ Triceps Punch-Out

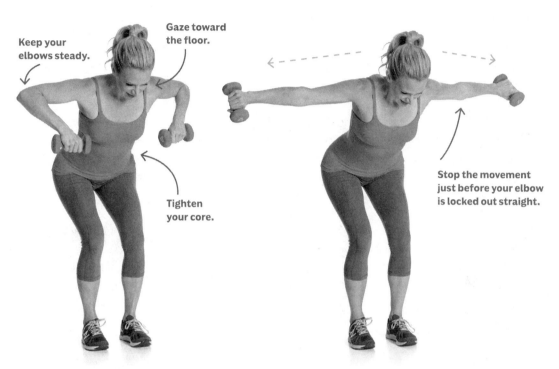

Keep your elbows steady.

Gaze toward the floor.

Tighten your core.

Stop the movement just before your elbow is locked out straight.

>> Stand tall with your feet hip-width apart and your arms by your sides, holding a weight in each hand. Keeping your back flat and abs engaged, hinge forward at your hips, arms hanging toward the floor with palms facing your body. Draw your elbows to shoulder height; this is your starting position. Keeping the upper arm steady, straighten your elbows to punch the weights back and up behind you. Pause for moment, then reverse the movement back to the starting position.

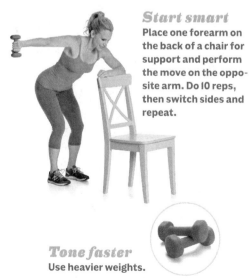

Start smart
Place one forearm on the back of a chair for support and perform the move on the opposite arm. Do 10 reps, then switch sides and repeat.

Tone faster
Use heavier weights.

④ Pull-Apart Bands

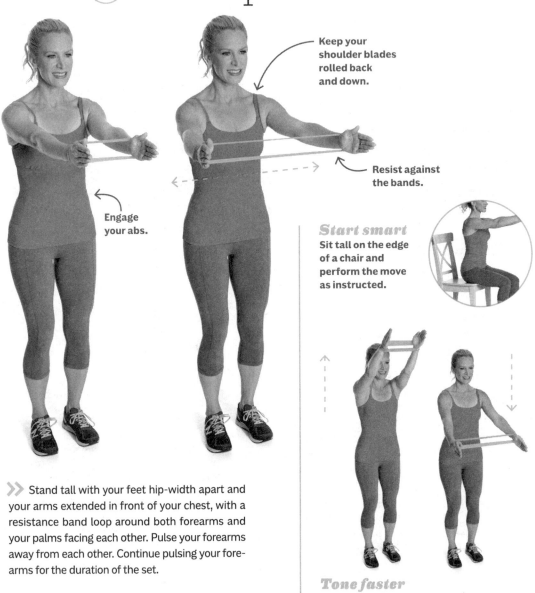

Keep your shoulder blades rolled back and down.

Resist against the bands.

Engage your abs.

Start smart
Sit tall on the edge of a chair and perform the move as instructed.

≫ Stand tall with your feet hip-width apart and your arms extended in front of your chest, with a resistance band loop around both forearms and your palms facing each other. Pulse your forearms away from each other. Continue pulsing your forearms for the duration of the set.

Tone faster
For an added challenge, slowly raise your arms up and down in front of your body as you pulse your forearms apart.

⑤ Chair Dip

>> Sit tall on the edge of a sturdy chair with your hands grasping the seat on either side of your butt and your feet flat on the floor. Slide your butt off the chair seat and walk your feet forward slightly, so your knees are directly over your ankles. Keeping your shoulders down, slowly bend your elbows back, lowering your butt toward the floor until your upper arms are nearly parallel to the floor. Hold for I second, then press back up.

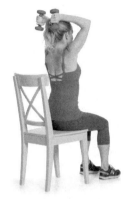

Start smart

If you can't put weight on your hands, do a seated triceps extension. Sit tall on the edge of a chair, holding one weight in each hand. Lift the weights over your head, positioning your elbows near your ears. Bending your elbows, slowly lower the weights behind your head. Hold for a second, then lift the weights back up.

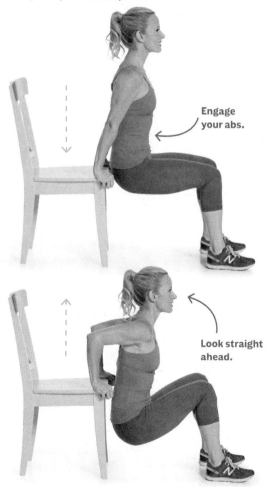

Engage your abs.

Look straight ahead.

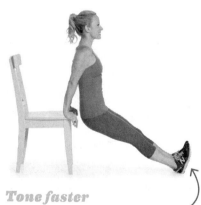

Tone faster

Walk your feet farther away from the chair, extending your legs and balancing on your heels.

BACK TO STRONG

Shed bra bulge and back fat faster with this 10-minute sculpting routine that targets every inch of your beautiful back. These moves will also help stabilize your spine, improve your posture, and help you reduce the risk of back pain. All you need is a pair of hand weights.

How to do it: Perform each exercise for 20 seconds, and rest for 10 seconds as you transition to the next move. Do the circuit 4 times.

① Single/Single/ Double Bent-Over Rows

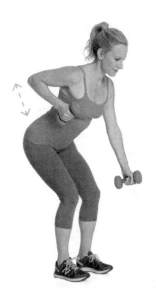
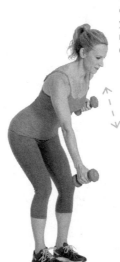

Check your form in a mirror to ensure your back is flat. When your back is rounded, you're not able to squeeze your shoulder blades together.

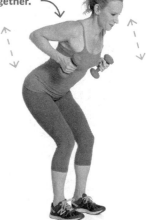

>> Stand tall with your feet shoulder-width apart, your knees slightly bent, and your arms at your sides, holding a weight in each hand. Bend over from the hips until your back is almost parallel to the floor. Pull the right weight to your shoulder, then lower. Pull the left weight to your shoulder, then lower. Now pull both weights to your shoulders, squeezing your shoulder blades together. Pause, then lower the weights.

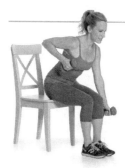

Start smart
Sit on the edge of a sturdy chair and perform the move as instructed.

Tone faster
Increase your weight. Don't be afraid to go heavy here!

② T Raise

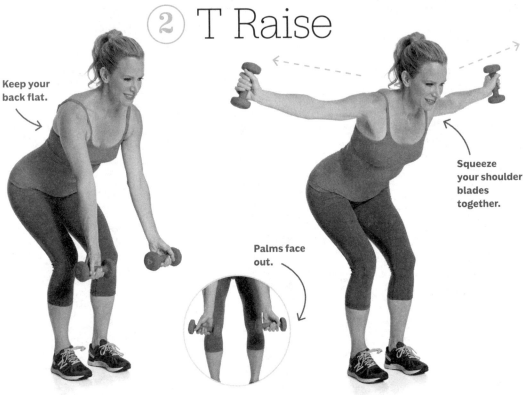

Keep your back flat.

Squeeze your shoulder blades together.

Palms face out.

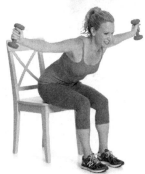

>> Stand tall with your feet shoulder-width apart, your knees slightly bent, and your arms at your sides, holding a weight in each hand. Bend over from the hips until your back is almost parallel to the floor. Extend your arms toward floor, palms facing forward. This is your starting position. Raise your arms out to the sides, forming a T, squeezing your shoulder blades together. Slowly reverse to the starting position.

Start smart
Sit tall on the edge of a chair and perform the move as instructed.

Tone faster
Use a heavier weight.

③ Knee Pushup with a Leg Raise

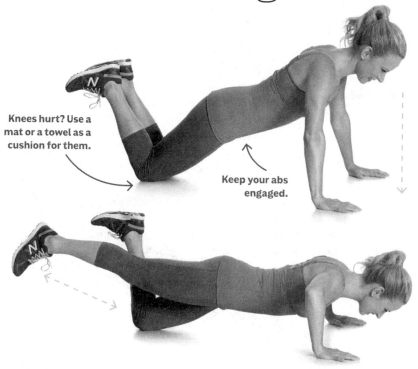

Knees hurt? Use a mat or a towel as a cushion for them.

Keep your abs engaged.

>> Kneel on the floor with your hands directly beneath your shoulders and your legs bent so that your body is in a straight line from your head to your knees. Lower your chest to the floor as you extend one leg behind you at hip height. Hold for a second, return your knee to the floor, then push back up. Alternate extended legs with each rep.

Start smart
Omit the leg raise and do a regular knee pushup.

Tone faster
Do a full pushup with both legs extended.

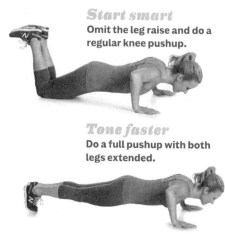

④ Plank Row

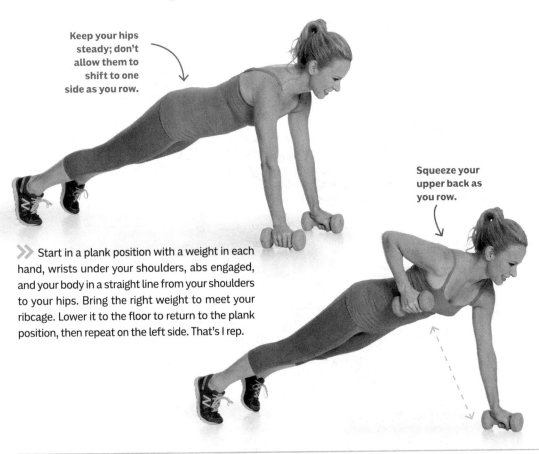

Keep your hips steady; don't allow them to shift to one side as you row.

Squeeze your upper back as you row.

>> Start in a plank position with a weight in each hand, wrists under your shoulders, abs engaged, and your body in a straight line from your shoulders to your hips. Bring the right weight to meet your ribcage. Lower it to the floor to return to the plank position, then repeat on the left side. That's I rep.

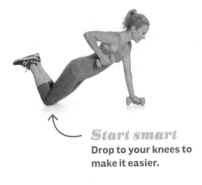

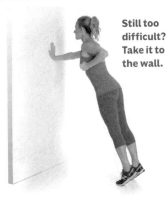

Still too difficult? Take it to the wall.

Start smart
Drop to your knees to make it easier.

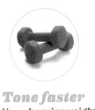

Tone faster
Use a heavier weight.

⑤ Superwoman

» Lie on your belly with your legs and arms extended. Simultaneously raise your arms, chest, and legs off the floor and hold for I second. Slowly lower back to the starting position.

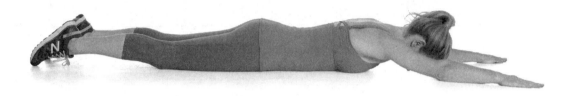

Squeeze your back to lift your body off the floor.

Keep your gaze down.

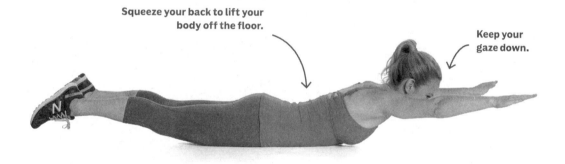

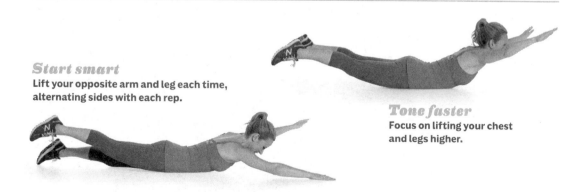

Start smart
Lift your opposite arm and leg each time, alternating sides with each rep.

Tone faster
Focus on lifting your chest and legs higher.

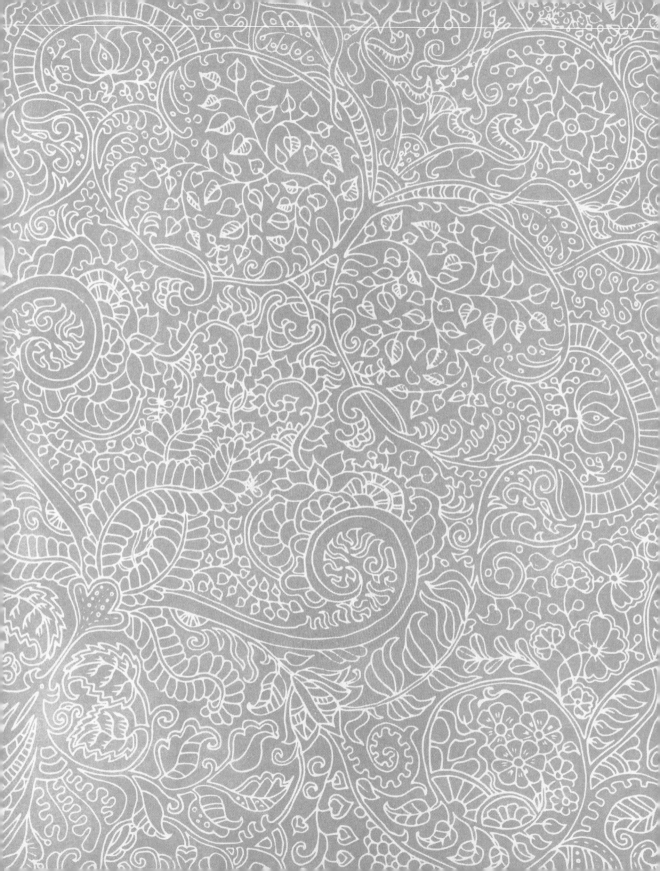

TONE ZONE
BELLY

If you're frustrated by stubborn abs that refuse to change, these 10-minute routines will help you strengthen and reshape your core in just minutes a day. They work by targeting your deepest belly muscles with a combination of light weights, bands, and your body weight. Stick with them, and you'll start to see and feel a difference in just a few weeks. "I loved feeling my core become stronger each day," says Lori Lowell, 59, who lost 6.5 inches off her abs in just 8 weeks.

FLAT AND FIRM ABS

Build a strong, slender core with these metabolism-revving tummy toners. All you need is a mat or a carpeted surface. If you want to kick up the calorie burn, grab a hand weight.

How to do it: Perform each exercise for 20 seconds, and rest for 10 seconds as you transition to the next move. Do the circuit 4 times.

① Tabletop Crunch

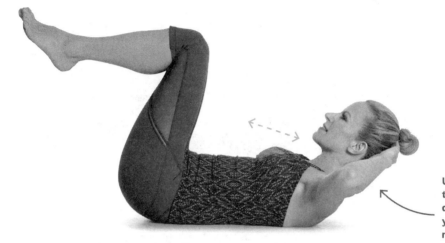

Use your abs to crunch up; don't pull on your head or neck.

» Lie on your back with your knees bent at 90 degrees and raised over your hips, as if your heels were resting on a tabletop. Without pulling on your neck, exhale and lift your shoulders and chest slightly off the mat. Slowly reverse the move.

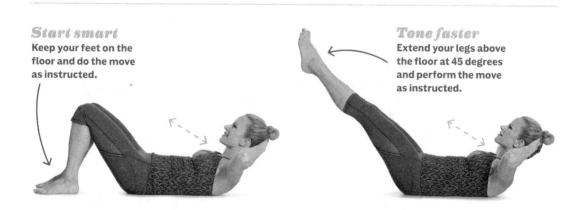

Start smart
Keep your feet on the floor and do the move as instructed.

Tone faster
Extend your legs above the floor at 45 degrees and perform the move as instructed.

② Single/Single/Double-Leg Drop

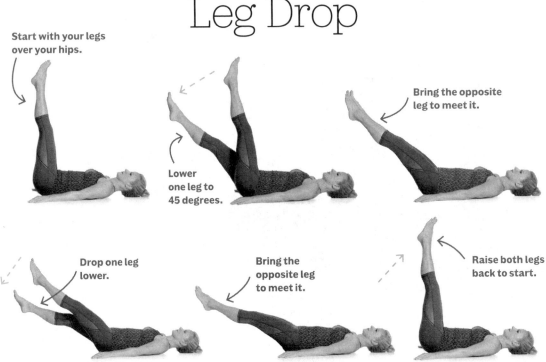

Start with your legs over your hips.

Lower one leg to 45 degrees.

Bring the opposite leg to meet it.

Drop one leg lower.

Bring the opposite leg to meet it.

Raise both legs back to start.

➤➤ Lie on your back with your legs extended over your hips and your arms by your sides. Pull your belly in and press your lower back into the floor. This is your starting position. Lower your right leg to 45 degrees. Pause, then lower your left leg to meet your right leg. Pause, then lower your right leg to a 2-inch hover above the floor. Pause, then bring your left leg to meet it. Pause, then raise both legs back to start. Repeat, starting with the left leg. Continue alternating the starting leg with each rep.

Start smart
Bend your knees to tabletop position and do toe taps instead. Alternate dropping the left foot to the floor, then the right.

Tone faster
Place your hands behind your head and curl your chest and shoulders off the floor. Perform the move as instructed.

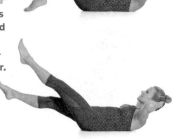

③ V Crunch

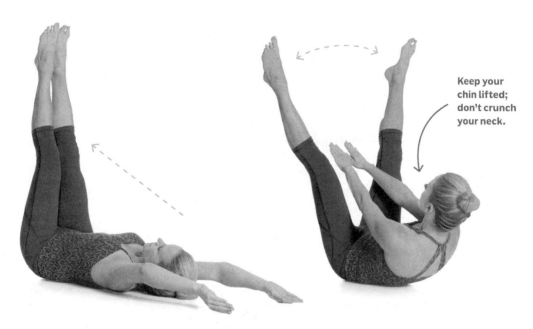

Keep your chin lifted; don't crunch your neck.

≫ Lie on your back with your legs extended over your hips and your arms extended on the floor overhead. Use your abs to lift your upper back off the floor and lower legs out to the sides, reaching your hands between your legs. Slowly reverse the move back to start.

Start smart
Bend your knees to the tabletop position and tap your hands to your knees.

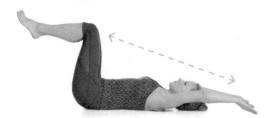

Tone faster
Hold one weight with both hands. Perform the move as instructed.

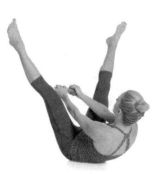

④ Flutter Kick

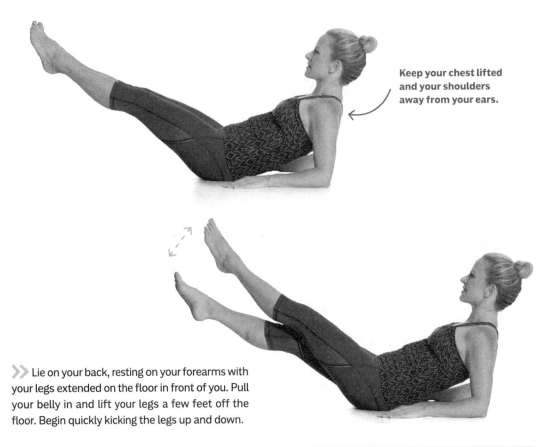

Keep your chest lifted and your shoulders away from your ears.

>> Lie on your back, resting on your forearms with your legs extended on the floor in front of you. Pull your belly in and lift your legs a few feet off the floor. Begin quickly kicking the legs up and down.

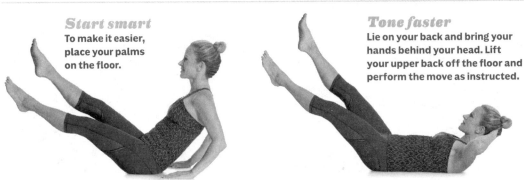

Start smart
To make it easier, place your palms on the floor.

Tone faster
Lie on your back and bring your hands behind your head. Lift your upper back off the floor and perform the move as instructed.

⑤ Plank Rocks

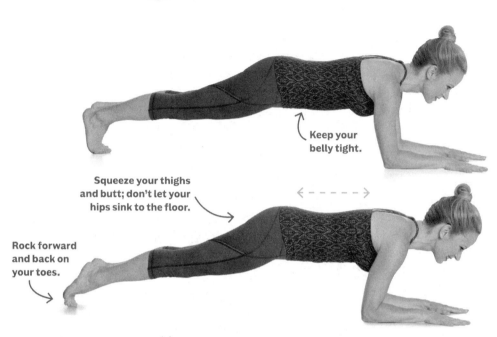

Keep your belly tight.

Squeeze your thighs and butt; don't let your hips sink to the floor.

Rock forward and back on your toes.

>> Start in a forearm plank position with your elbows under your shoulders, keeping your hips and shoulders in a straight line. Gently rock your torso forward, then back toward your heels. Continue rocking, keeping your entire core tight and strong during the whole movement.

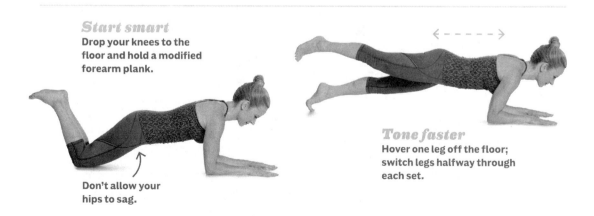

Start smart
Drop your knees to the floor and hold a modified forearm plank.

Don't allow your hips to sag.

Tone faster
Hover one leg off the floor; switch legs halfway through each set.

DEEP CORE

This 10-minute routine combines highly effective Pilates work with essential corrective exercises to help you reactivate belly muscles quickly and gently. The result: a tight, toned core that will support your every move and reduce the risk of back pain.

How to do it: Perform each exercise for 20 seconds, and rest for 10 seconds as you transition to the next move. Do the circuit 4 times.

① Dead Bug to Reverse Crunch

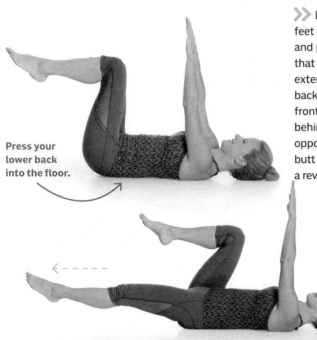

Press your lower back into the floor.

>> Lie on your back with your knees bent and your feet flat on the floor. Pull your belly to your spine and press your lower back into the floor. Keeping that position, raise your knees over your hips and extend your arms over your chest. Keeping your back pressed into the floor, extend your left leg in front of you to a 2-inch hover and your right arm behind your head. Return to start and repeat on opposite side. Now, pull your belly in and lift your butt and hips a few inches off the floor to perform a reverse crunch. That's 1 rep.

Extend your opposite arm and leg.

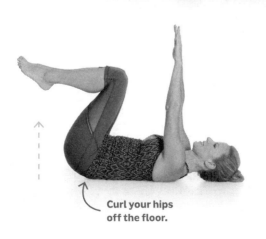

Curl your hips off the floor.

Start smart
Keep your knees bent.

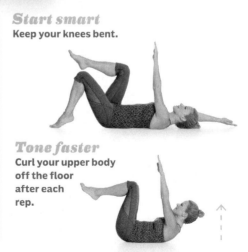

Tone faster
Curl your upper body off the floor after each rep.

② Windmill

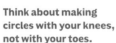

Think about making circles with your knees, not with your toes.

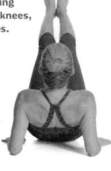

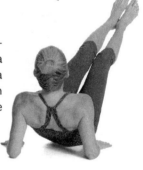

>> Lie on your back with your weight on your forearms, your knees bent and lifted over your hips in a tabletop position. Leading with your knees, make a circle with your legs in a clockwise motion. When you return to the starting position, repeat the circle in the opposite direction.

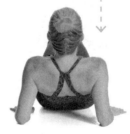

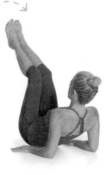

Start smart
Keep your circles small and controlled; increase your range of motion as the core becomes stronger.

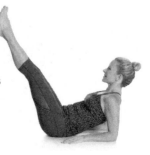

Tone faster
Extend your legs, keeping your heels together, and perform the move as instructed.

③ Ab Tuck

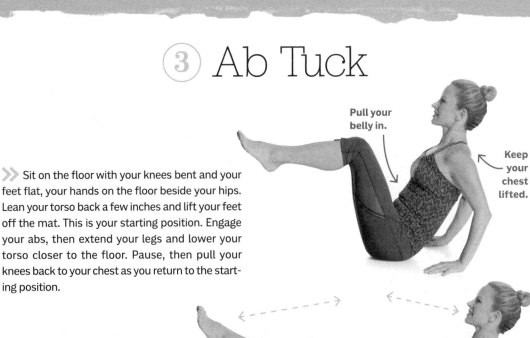

Pull your belly in.

Keep your chest lifted.

>> Sit on the floor with your knees bent and your feet flat, your hands on the floor beside your hips. Lean your torso back a few inches and lift your feet off the mat. This is your starting position. Engage your abs, then extend your legs and lower your torso closer to the floor. Pause, then pull your knees back to your chest as you return to the starting position.

If you feel this in your lower back, don't lower the legs or torso as far to the floor.

Start smart

Sit on the edge of a sturdy chair. Hold onto the seat and lean your torso back slightly to raise your knees toward your chest. Tap your feet to the floor, then raise your knees back to start.

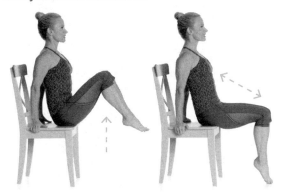

Tone faster

Place a 2- to 5-pound weight between your feet and perform the move as instructed.

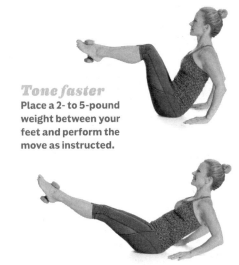

④ Bird Dog

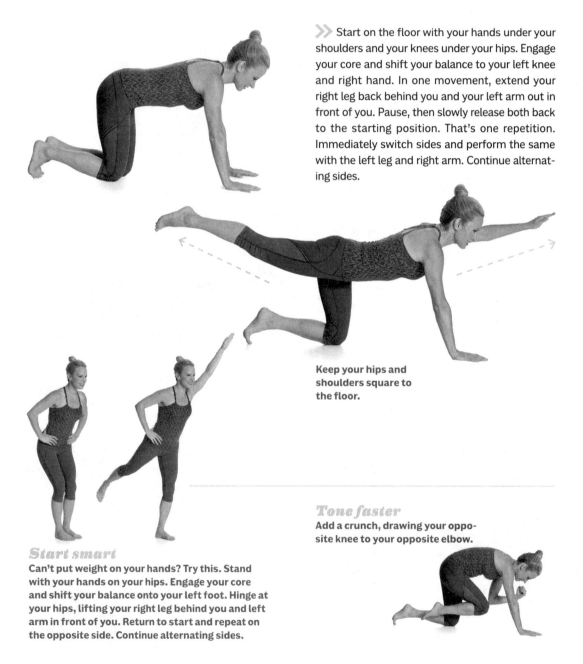

>> Start on the floor with your hands under your shoulders and your knees under your hips. Engage your core and shift your balance to your left knee and right hand. In one movement, extend your right leg back behind you and your left arm out in front of you. Pause, then slowly release both back to the starting position. That's one repetition. Immediately switch sides and perform the same with the left leg and right arm. Continue alternating sides.

Keep your hips and shoulders square to the floor.

Tone faster
Add a crunch, drawing your opposite knee to your opposite elbow.

Start smart
Can't put weight on your hands? Try this. Stand with your hands on your hips. Engage your core and shift your balance onto your left foot. Hinge at your hips, lifting your right leg behind you and left arm in front of you. Return to start and repeat on the opposite side. Continue alternating sides.

⑤ Side Plank Sweep

>> Start in a forearm side plank on your left arm, feet staggered, right arm extended over your shoulder. Sweep your right arm down and under your ribcage, rotating your torso. Sweep your right arm back to start. Continue for 20 seconds, then switch sides and repeat for another 20 seconds.

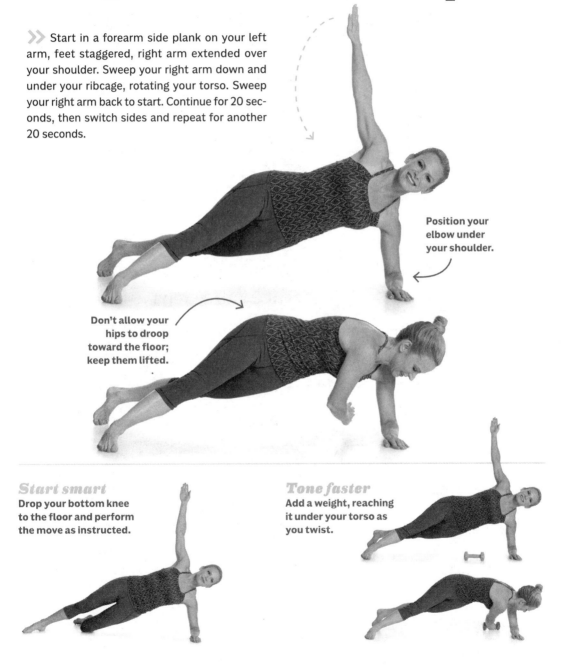

Position your elbow under your shoulder.

Don't allow your hips to droop toward the floor; keep them lifted.

Start smart
Drop your bottom knee to the floor and perform the move as instructed.

Tone faster
Add a weight, reaching it under your torso as you twist.

TUMMY LOVE

Ready for a belly-firming challenge that will slim your middle in record time? It's time to add resistance band loops to these incredibly effective ab moves. In addition to isolating your core, the bands will help you score some extra hip and thigh toning.

How to do it: Perform each exercise for 20 seconds, and rest for 10 seconds as you transition to the next move. Do the circuit 4 times.

① Butterfly Band Crunch

Keep tension on the band; activating your glutes helps you to press your lower back into the floor so you can isolate your abs.

Don't pull on your neck. Keep your chin lifted.

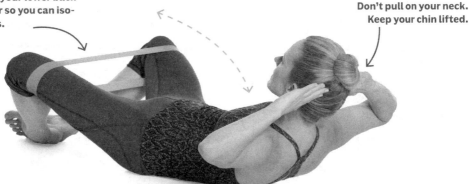

>> Sit on the floor with your knees bent and feet flat, a resistance band loop around your thighs (positioned slightly above your knees). Lie on your back and bring the soles of your feet together, allowing your knees to drop to the sides. Place your hands behind your head and crunch up and down, lifting your shoulders and chest off the floor.

Start smart
Omit the band and perform the move as instructed.

Tone faster
Hold a weight with both hands at your chest to increase the challenge.

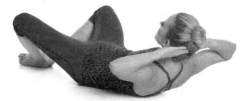

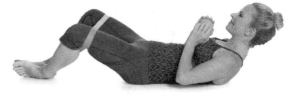

② Scissors

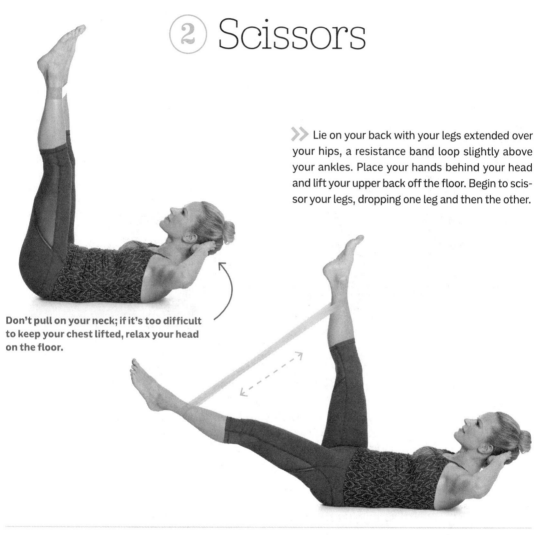

>> Lie on your back with your legs extended over your hips, a resistance band loop slightly above your ankles. Place your hands behind your head and lift your upper back off the floor. Begin to scissor your legs, dropping one leg and then the other.

Don't pull on your neck; if it's too difficult to keep your chest lifted, relax your head on the floor.

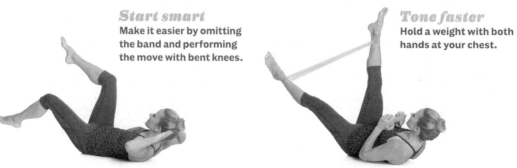

Start smart
Make it easier by omitting the band and performing the move with bent knees.

Tone faster
Hold a weight with both hands at your chest.

③ Leg Drops with Abduction

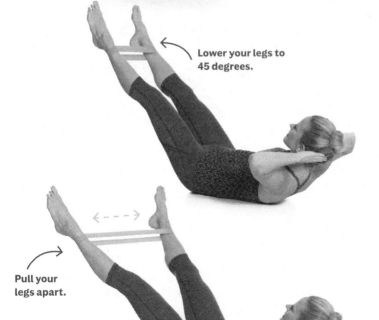

Start with your legs over your hips.

Lower your legs to 45 degrees.

Pull your legs apart.

>> Lie on your back with your legs extended over your hips and a resistance band loop slightly above your ankles. Place your hands behind your head and keep your shoulders lifted. Lower both legs down to about 45 degrees; hold the position and separate your legs. Bring them back to about hip-distance apart, then raise legs back to start.

Start smart

Omit the leg drop; keep your legs extended over your hips and perform the move as instructed.

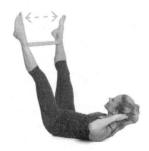

Tone faster

Hold a weight with both hands at your chest.

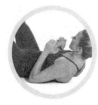

④ Band Bicycles

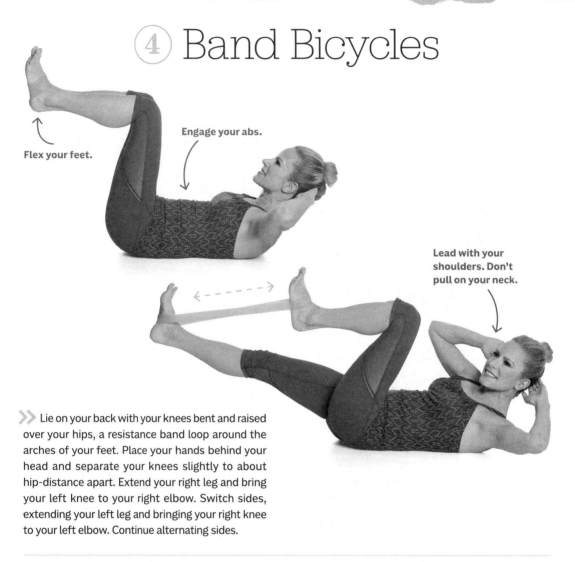

Flex your feet.

Engage your abs.

Lead with your shoulders. Don't pull on your neck.

>> Lie on your back with your knees bent and raised over your hips, a resistance band loop around the arches of your feet. Place your hands behind your head and separate your knees slightly to about hip-distance apart. Extend your right leg and bring your left knee to your right elbow. Switch sides, extending your left leg and bringing your right knee to your left elbow. Continue alternating sides.

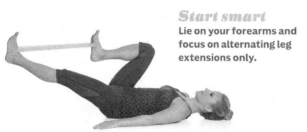

Start smart
Lie on your forearms and focus on alternating leg extensions only.

Tone faster
Increase your speed and band resistance.

⑤ Band Crunch

Flex your feet.

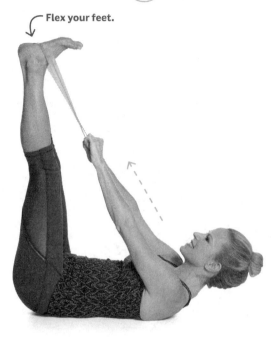

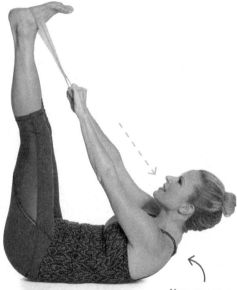

Use your core to lift your upper back. Don't use momentum.

» Lie on your back with your legs extended over your hips, a resistance band loop around the arches of the feet, holding the other end of the loop with both hands. Crunch your upper back off the floor and slowly lower back down, feeling the negative resistance of the band.

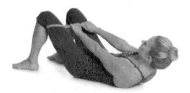

Start smart

Keep your feet flat on the floor and place the band around your thighs.

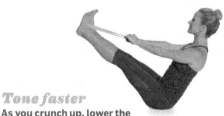

Tone faster

As you crunch up, lower the legs to 45 degrees, coming up into a boat pose. Pause, then rock back to start.

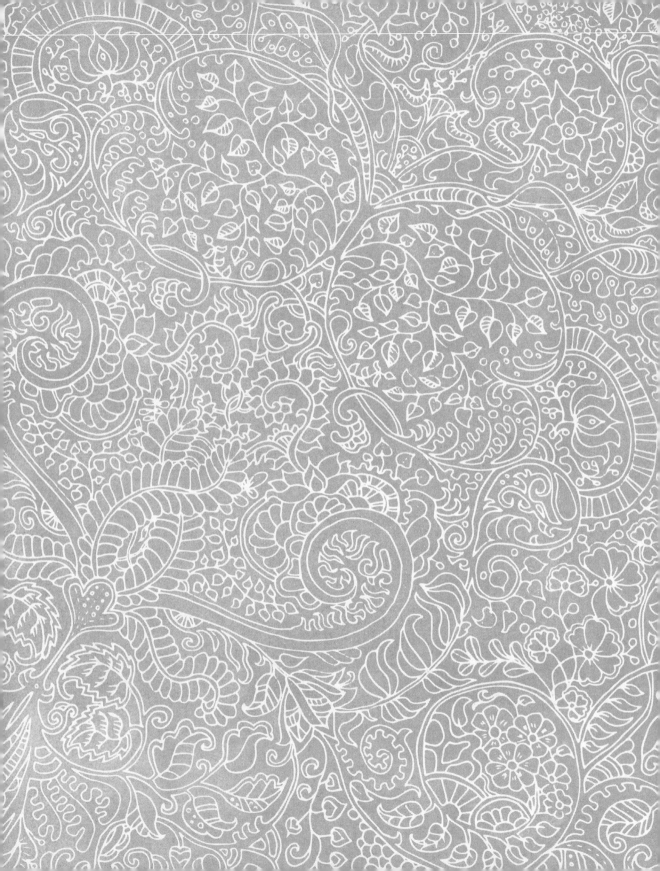

TOTAL BODY

It's time to tone and tighten every inch with these metabolism-driving combo moves. You'll kick up your calorie burn while sculpting your legs, arms, back, and belly. Don't be surprised by how quickly you break a sweat. "I used to think that I needed to work out for an hour for it to make an impact," says Sarah M., 33, who lost 18 pounds on the plan. "Now I know that 10 minutes really counts."

SIZZLE
AND
SCULPT

Lower-body toning meets upper-body firming in this calorie-igniting routine that builds lean, sexy muscle. Grab your weights, a resistance band loop, and a mat— and prepare to get sweaty.

How to do it: Do two rounds of Circuit I, then two rounds of Circuit 2. Perform each exercise for 40 seconds and rest for 20 seconds as you transition to the next move.

① Rainbow Side Bend

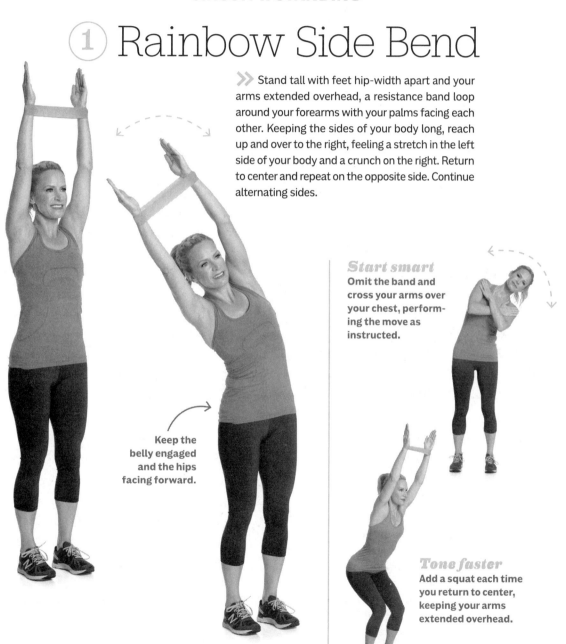

》 Stand tall with feet hip-width apart and your arms extended overhead, a resistance band loop around your forearms with your palms facing each other. Keeping the sides of your body long, reach up and over to the right, feeling a stretch in the left side of your body and a crunch on the right. Return to center and repeat on the opposite side. Continue alternating sides.

Keep the belly engaged and the hips facing forward.

Start smart
Omit the band and cross your arms over your chest, performing the move as instructed.

Tone faster
Add a squat each time you return to center, keeping your arms extended overhead.

② Lunge 'n' Pull

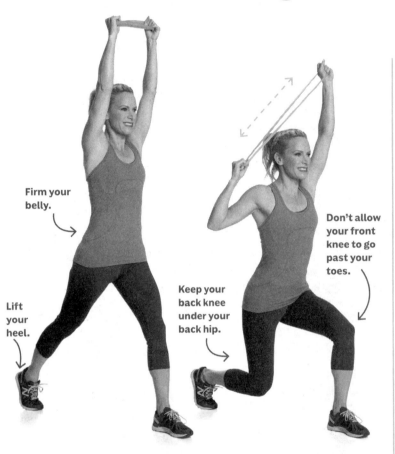

Firm your belly.

Lift your heel.

Keep your back knee under your back hip.

Don't allow your front knee to go past your toes.

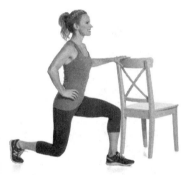

Start smart
Place one hand on the back of a chair and omit the pulldown.

>> Stand in a split stance with your right leg back and your left leg forward, arms extended overhead, with one end of a resistance band loop in each hand. Bend both of your knees to lower into a lunge as you pull your right elbow down toward your right shoulder. Your left arm remains steady and straight. Slowly reverse the move back to start. Continue for 20 seconds; switch sides and repeat for another 20 seconds.

Tone faster
Use a heavier band to increase the resistance.

③ Squat with Shoulder Squeeze

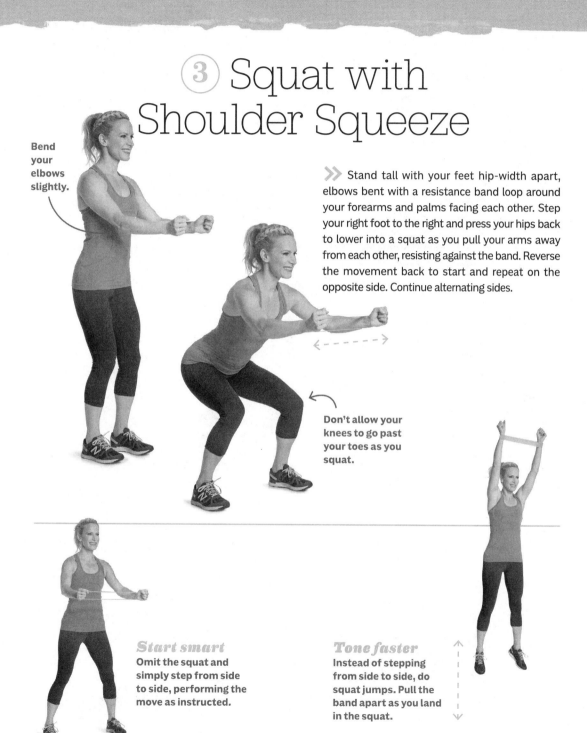

Bend your elbows slightly.

≫ Stand tall with your feet hip-width apart, elbows bent with a resistance band loop around your forearms and palms facing each other. Step your right foot to the right and press your hips back to lower into a squat as you pull your arms away from each other, resisting against the band. Reverse the movement back to start and repeat on the opposite side. Continue alternating sides.

Don't allow your knees to go past your toes as you squat.

Start smart
Omit the squat and simply step from side to side, performing the move as instructed.

Tone faster
Instead of stepping from side to side, do squat jumps. Pull the band apart as you land in the squat.

CIRCUIT 2: FLOOR

④ Plank Step-Outs

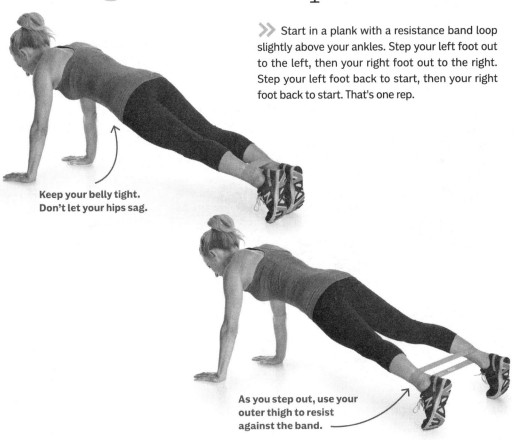

>> Start in a plank with a resistance band loop slightly above your ankles. Step your left foot out to the left, then your right foot out to the right. Step your left foot back to start, then your right foot back to start. That's one rep.

Keep your belly tight. Don't let your hips sag.

As you step out, use your outer thigh to resist against the band.

Start smart
To make it easier, drop to your forearms.

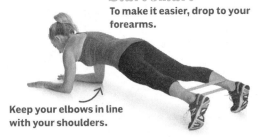

Keep your elbows in line with your shoulders.

Tone faster
Between each rep, drop to your knees and perform a triceps pushup.

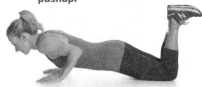

⑤ Side Plank Roll

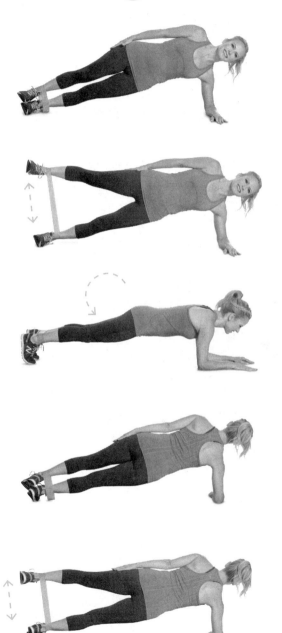

>> Start in a forearm side plank on your left side, with your legs extended and a resistance band loop around your ankles. Lift your right leg, keeping your foot flexed. Pause, then lower your leg back to start and roll your torso toward the floor, coming into a forearm plank with your elbows under your shoulders. Move into a side plank on your right forearm and lift your left leg. Pause, then lower your leg and return to forearm plank. Continue alternating sides with each rep.

Start smart

Do the move without a band. To make it even easier, omit the leg lift or just hold a modified forearm plank with your knees on the floor.

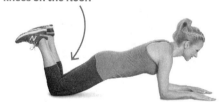

Tone faster

Use a heavier band to increase the resistance.

META BLAST

Turn back the clock on your body and metabolism with this muscle-building power circuit that torches calories and sculpts a strong, lean physique. All you need is a mat and a pair of hand weights.

How to do it: Do each move for 40 seconds, resting for 10 seconds as you transition to the Cardio Burst. Do the Cardio Burst for 20 seconds after each exercise, resting for 5 seconds before starting the next move. Do the circuit twice.

① Narrow Squat to Wide Squat

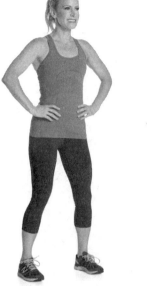
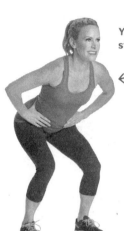
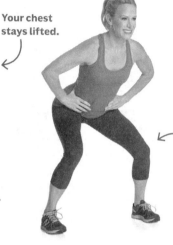

Your chest stays lifted.

Keep a deep bend in your knees as you move between squats.

>> Stand tall with your feet hip-width apart, abs engaged, and your hands on your hips. Step your right foot out to the right and lower into a wide squat. Straighten your legs halfway and step your right foot back to the start. Immediately lower into a narrow squat. Straighten your legs halfway and step your left leg to the left, lowering into a wider squat. Reverse the movement back to the start. Continue alternating between narrow and wide squats, alternating sides with each rep.

Start smart
Place your hands on the back of a chair and perform the move as instructed.

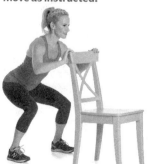

Tone faster
Hop from narrow to wide squats, omitting the side-to-side steps.

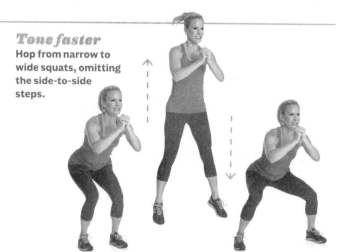

② Cardio Burst: Jack 'n' Press

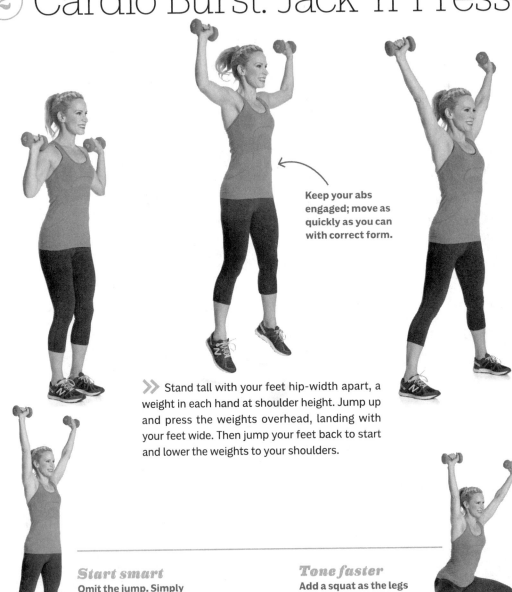

Keep your abs engaged; move as quickly as you can with correct form.

» Stand tall with your feet hip-width apart, a weight in each hand at shoulder height. Jump up and press the weights overhead, landing with your feet wide. Then jump your feet back to start and lower the weights to your shoulders.

Start smart
Omit the jump. Simply alternate tapping one foot out to the side, then the other, as you press the weights overhead.

Tone faster
Add a squat as the legs go wide, hopping the feet back together as you lower the weights back to your shoulders.

③ Sumo Squat with a Biceps Curl

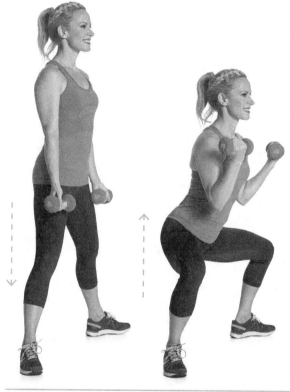

>> Stand with your feet wider than shoulder-width apart, your toes turned out slightly, and your arms hanging in front of body, with one weight in each hand. Bend your knees and lower your hips into a sumo squat, curling the weights toward your shoulders. Reverse the move back to start.

Keep your knees tracking over your toes.

Repeat Cardio Burst

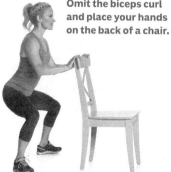

Start smart
Omit the biceps curl and place your hands on the back of a chair.

Tone faster
Do sumo squat jumps. Jump your feet apart, landing in a squat as you curl the weights to your shoulders. Jump back to start.

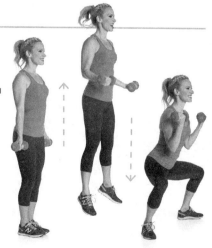

④ Plank Hops

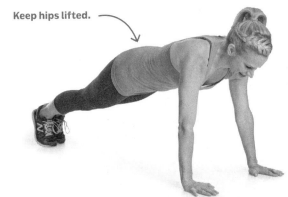

Keep hips lifted.

>> Begin in a plank position, your wrists in line with your shoulders. Bend your knees and hop your feet to the right. Pause for a moment, and then repeat, hopping your feet to the left. Continue alternating sides with each hop.

Repeat Cardio Burst, page 118

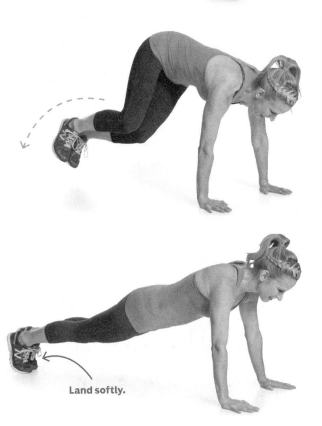

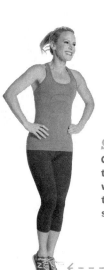

Start smart
Can't get down on the floor? Stand with your feet together and hop side to side.

Land softly.

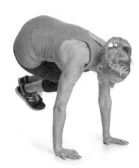

Tone faster
Hop side to side without pausing.

⑤ Arms Up Partial Situp

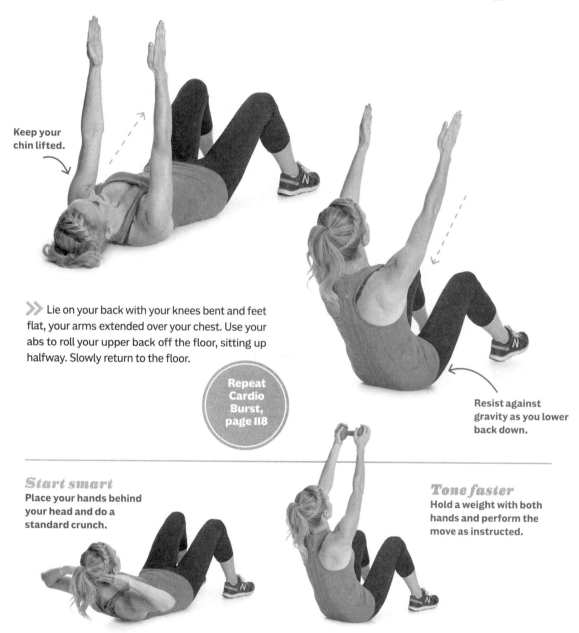

Keep your chin lifted.

» Lie on your back with your knees bent and feet flat, your arms extended over your chest. Use your abs to roll your upper back off the floor, sitting up halfway. Slowly return to the floor.

Repeat Cardio Burst, page 118

Resist against gravity as you lower back down.

Start smart
Place your hands behind your head and do a standard crunch.

Tone faster
Hold a weight with both hands and perform the move as instructed.

TORCH TO TONE

These fat-burning moves use nothing more than your own bodyweight to spike heart rate, incinerate calories, and carve lean, beautiful muscle. Bonus: They're easily modified, so you can work smart and still see results.

How to do it: Do each move for 40 seconds, resting for 10 seconds as you transition to the Push Move. Do the Push Move for 20 seconds after each exercise, resting for 5 seconds before starting the next move. Do the circuit twice.

① Half Jack with a Knee Lift

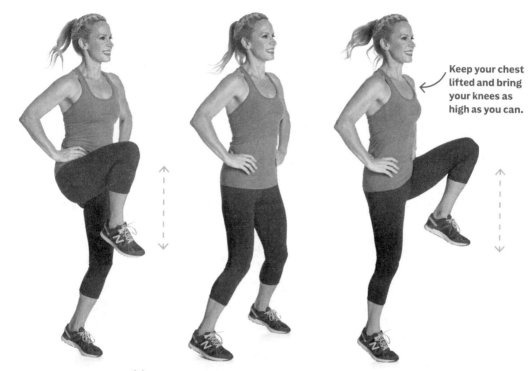

Keep your chest lifted and bring your knees as high as you can.

» Stand tall with your feet together and your hands on your hips. Hop your feet apart and raise one knee toward your chest. Reverse the move and repeat on the opposite side.

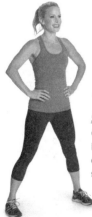

Start smart
Omit the knee raise. If the jack is too difficult, simply step side to side.

Tone faster
Do a sumo squat jump. Start as instructed, then jump your legs wider than hip-width apart and lower into a squat. Jump back to start.

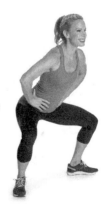

② Push Move: Long Jump

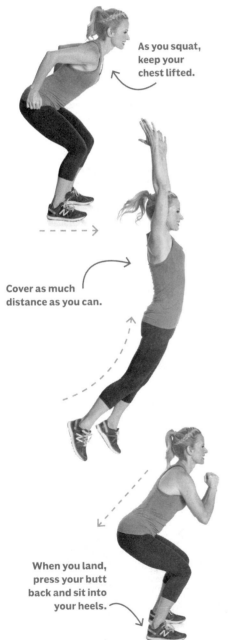

As you squat, keep your chest lifted.

Cover as much distance as you can.

When you land, press your butt back and sit into your heels.

>> Stand tall with your feet hip-width apart and your abs engaged. Bend your knees and swing your arms behind you, then swing your arms overhead and jump forward as far as you can with both feet. Land softly in a squat, keeping your knees behind your toes. Stand up and quickly jog backward to your starting position. Repeat.

Start smart
Do a regular squat with your hands on the back of a chair for balance. March in place for a few seconds between squats.

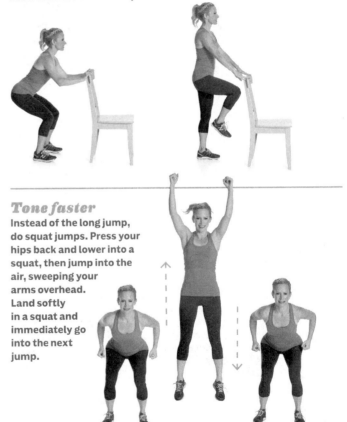

Tone faster
Instead of the long jump, do squat jumps. Press your hips back and lower into a squat, then jump into the air, sweeping your arms overhead. Land softly in a squat and immediately go into the next jump.

③ Inchworm

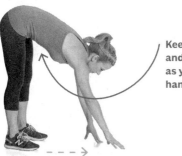

>> Stand tall with your feet hip-width apart. Hinge at your hips and fold forward, bringing your hands to the floor (bend your knees if needed). Walk your hands forward into a plank, then quickly walk your hands back to your feet and stand, returning to the starting position.

Repeat the Push Move

Keep your abs and core strong as you walk your hands out.

Start smart

Start kneeling with your palms on the floor and directly in front of your knees (your back will be slightly rounded). Walk your hands forward until you are in a modified plank. Walk your hands back to your knees. Repeat.

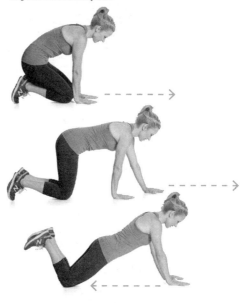

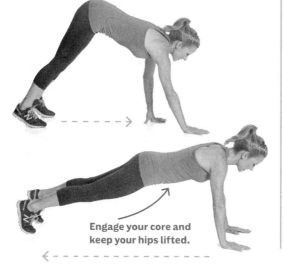

Engage your core and keep your hips lifted.

Tone faster

Add a triceps pushup each time you walk out to a plank.

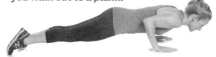

④ Plank to Shin Tap

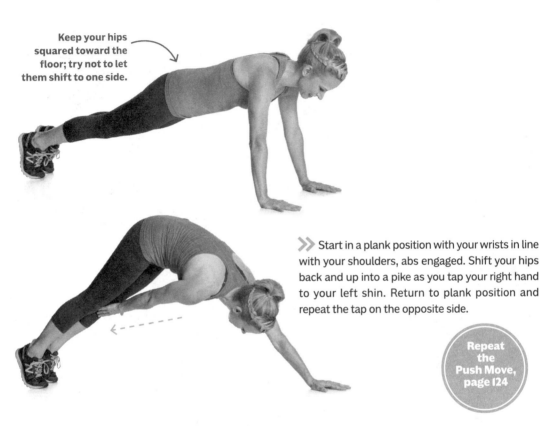

Keep your hips squared toward the floor; try not to let them shift to one side.

>> Start in a plank position with your wrists in line with your shoulders, abs engaged. Shift your hips back and up into a pike as you tap your right hand to your left shin. Return to plank position and repeat the tap on the opposite side.

Repeat the Push Move, page 124

Start smart
Do a modified plank with your knees on the floor; alternate tapping your opposite hand to your opposite thigh.

Tone faster
Perform the move as instructed, but tap your hand to your ankle instead of your calf.

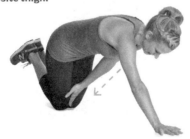

⑤ Sprinter Situp

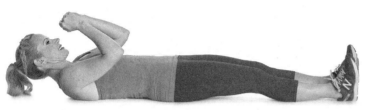

>> Lie on your back with your legs extended. Engage your core to lift your torso off the floor, drawing your right knee to your left elbow. Reverse the move back to the starting position and quickly repeat on the opposite side. Continue alternating sides with each rep.

Engage your obliques as you bring your opposite knee to your opposite elbow.

Repeat the Push Move, page 124

Start smart
Do bicycle crunches instead.

Tone faster
Perform the move as instructed, but keep your legs slightly lifted off the floor.

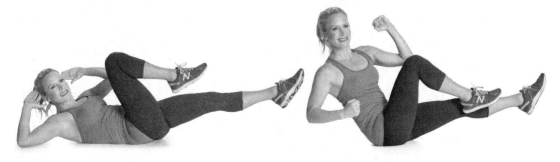

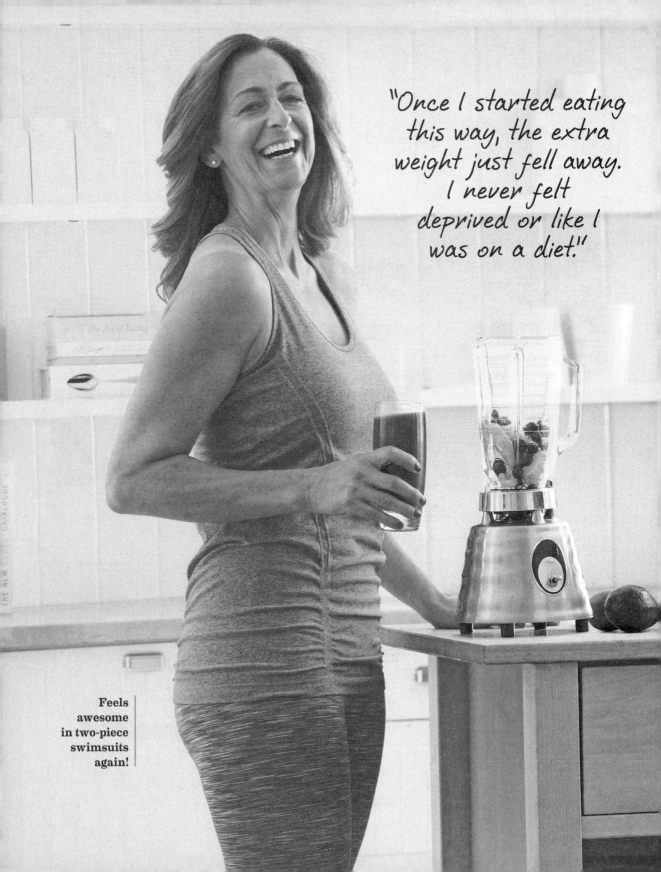

"Once I started eating this way, the extra weight just fell away. I never felt deprived or like I was on a diet."

Feels awesome in two-piece swimsuits again!

Anne Marie Russo

AGE:	**53**
POUNDS LOST:	**26**
INCHES LOST:	**14.25**

Anne Marie Russo had always loved summer. Every year, she'd spend hours by the pool and at the beach with her husband and their three children. "I always wore a two-piece," says the stay-at-home mom. "Even after three pregnancies, I could still pull it off." When Anne Marie turned 50, though, everything changed. Suddenly, her tall, naturally thin body started to hold on to every extra calorie. "It was frustrating to see my middle getting thicker and to see myself creeping up in sizes," she recalls. "It was bumming me out and making me feel awful about myself." She tried to shrink her growing waist by skipping breakfast and pushing herself through three intense boot-camp classes a week, but nothing seemed to work. "It was like I hit a wall. No matter what I tried, I felt like my body wasn't changing."

When she realized she no longer felt comfortable in the two-piece swimsuits she loved, Anne Marie knew she needed to make a change. "I hated the idea of wearing a one-piece; it just made me feel older and not as attractive," she says. "I thought, if I don't do something now to change the way I'm eating and exercising, then I'm only going to get heavier."

When Anne Marie heard about the *Fit in 10: Slim & Strong–for Life!* program, she was excited to try it. "The idea of being strong and lean for life really appealed to me," says Anne Marie. "My kids are almost out of the house, and I want to have the health and energy to enjoy this next stage of my life with my husband."

So Anne Marie started following the Fit in 10 program. At first, as her body adjusted to clean eating, she admits she felt a little irritable. "My body was used to having a lot more sugar," she says. "But once I started reading labels, it made me think, *What the heck had I been eating?*" Within a few weeks of eating clean, Anne Marie's taste buds began to change. "I actually really started to enjoy eating this way," she says.

The 10-minute routines also made Anne Marie a consistent exerciser. "There wasn't a day that I missed a workout," she says. And that little bit of commitment had big payoffs.

Soon Anne Marie was seeing changes in her body. "My arms were stronger and more defined, and my belly started to shrink," says Anne Marie, who lost nearly 16 pounds in 8 weeks. Before starting the program, she had trouble getting through exercise without feeling winded. "Once I started eating healthier and doing the Fit in 10 routines, I could push myself a lot harder. I had so much more energy."

Now, Anne Marie is down 26 pounds and back in her two-piece suits. "Fit in 10 was the right thing for me at the right time," she says. "The program showed me that healthy food can taste delicious. I definitely want to continue eating and exercising this way."

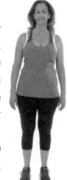

Why Anne Marie Loves Fit in 10

IT HELPS YOU DROP INCHES FAST. "I feel much better in my clothes. There was a pair of jeans that I was just squeezing into, and they looked horrible around my waist. Now, I could wear a crop top if I wanted to—they fit so much better!"

◀ BEFORE

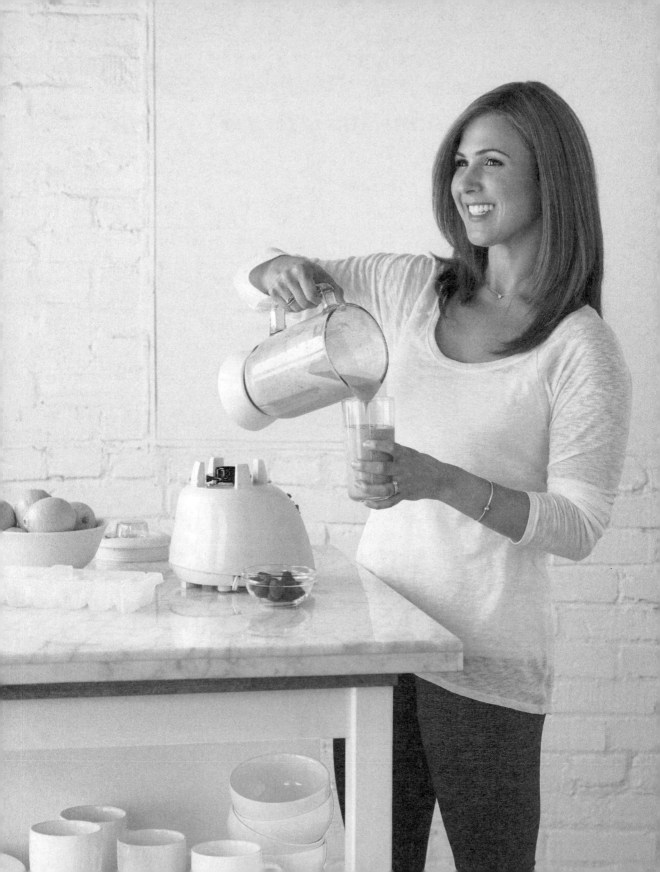

6

Quick Tricks to Go Clean and Lean

Ever go on a diet and it doesn't just make you feel awful, it makes everyone else around you miserable, too? The first (and last) time I ever did one of those silly juice cleanses, I convinced my husband that he needed to do it with me. While he magically seemed to be able to function on cucumber juice and spicy "lemonade," I basically turned into a crazy person. After thinking of nothing more than my intense desire to chew *something* all day, I'd come home from work, slam back the liquid "dinner" that was supposed to be making me feel great but was only turning me into a hangry monster, and climb into bed at 7 p.m. just so I wouldn't have to stand in my kitchen fantasizing

about the real food I'd rather be eating. Needless to say, it wasn't great for our relationship and by day 3, both of us were happy when I called it quits on the self-imposed misery.

That unpleasant experience underscored how much I appreciate good food and what a joy it gives me to sit down and savor a meal. Food is one of the best parts of life, and it's meant to be enjoyed—even on days when you have only a few minutes to throw together a couple of simple, fresh ingredients. That's why the Fit in 10 approach isn't about dieting. It's about making clean eating so quick, easy, and delicious that each bite feels like a reward while you up your energy and drop stubborn pounds. And with a few tips, tricks, and shortcuts, it's totally doable, even when you're pressed for time.

What Clean Eating Is All About

Think about the last time you bit into a strawberry that was perfectly sweet and juicy. Maybe you didn't grow it or pick it yourself, but other than the packing and transportation process that brought it to your local market, it was in its unadulterated, natural state (hopefully organic, or at least well washed). It wasn't packed with added sugar or sodium or preservatives. It didn't originate in a lab, and it still contained a healthy mix of antioxidants and fiber. Whether you realized it or not, you were eating clean at that moment.

Simply put, clean eating means avoiding as many packaged and highly processed foods as possible and opting for real, honest food instead. Basically, you'll eat more like your ancestors ate: closer to the earth.

This doesn't mean that you need to start a vegetable garden or raise your own chickens. While I love the idea of harvesting my own tomatoes or listening to hens clucking happily as I gather the eggs for a morning omelet, it's just not realistic for my busy life. (I also didn't inherit my mom's green thumb and think of weeding as a punishment.) Luckily, with the right know-how and a few simple shortcuts, clean eating can be as effortless as you need it to be, with many of the meals provided for you in Chapter 7 clocking in at no more than 10 minutes. Once you start to eat this way,

you'll realize how much better clean food tastes—and how much better you feel when you avoid the processed junk.

Why Eat Clean?

IT'S EASY AND ENJOYABLE. That's right, it's not a diet. Clean eating doesn't require you to blacklist entire food groups or to go crazy counting calories or points. That's why many people (including me and our Fit in 10 test panelists) find it possible to eat this way not just for a few weeks or months—but for life. We've adopted it as our baseline; an effortless lifestyle that naturally helps us—and soon, you—stay at a healthy weight. That's because eating this way makes you feel energized, satisfied, and happy—the exact opposite of how most diets make you feel (tired, starved, and miserable). "I had been on diets and cleanses in the past that were impossible to stick with long-term, but eating clean is totally possible to maintain," says Fit in 10 panelist Kimberlee Auerbach Berlin. "It makes me feel good about myself."

Sure, you'll be avoiding refined junk, but after a while you won't even want to eat that stuff. I know it can seem hard to believe. I remember when I first heard the concept of clean eating and the idea of never digging my hand into a box of Goldfish crackers seemed impossible. But as I started filling my plate with more whole, natural foods, my desire for the processed foods and snacks I used to think of as acceptable was no longer appetizing. Now, my body seriously craves whole foods. Rather than feeling like I *should* eat them, they're the foods I *want* to eat. When I want something sweet, I'll usually reach for nature's candy—cantaloupe, watermelon, strawberries, or whatever fruit is in season. If I'm really in the mood for ice cream or brownies, I'll whip up a quick and simple clean dessert like Raspberry Frozen Yogurt on page 252 made with whole ingredients that taste amazing—and doesn't leave me feeling bloated and full of regret. (For more ideas, see the snack recipes on pages 245 through 262). Do I ever have processed foods? Of course, but I'm always so, so happy to go back to eating clean at my next meal or snack. Because the more you eat clean, the better natural foods taste.

IT SLASHES ADDED SUGAR. Sugar used to be a once-in-a-while treat: cake on birthdays or ice cream after the softball team scored an important win. Now, it has infiltrated everything from cereals to yogurt to spaghetti sauce. Research shows that the average American now consumes a staggering 130 pounds of added sugar a year. That's nearly 22 teaspoons each day, which is nearly four times the American Heart Association's recommended limit.[1] When we eat that much sweet stuff, it's no wonder that our pants get tight. Not only is sugar full of empty calories, it also increases production of the fat-storage hormone insulin. The more insulin you produce, the hungrier you are

and the harder it is to lose weight and keep it off.[2] So by choosing clean, whole foods whenever possible and making smarter choices when buying packaged foods, you'll crush cravings and trim the extra calories without even really noticing they're gone.

Not so sure you can part with the sweet stuff? Consider this: When healthy men and women swapped their processed, sugar-filled diets for clean ones, they naturally started to prefer the taste of less-sweet foods, according to a 2016 study published in the *American Journal of Clinical Nutrition*.[3] Within 1 month of following a new diet, they found low-sugar pudding to taste much sweeter than it did to people who continued to eat the standard sugar-laced diet. What's really cool is that even though the pudding had less sugar, the clean eaters found it to be just as pleasant as the sweet foods they ate prior to making the change.

"I'm someone who loves sweet foods—I used to put four packets of sugar in my coffee—so cutting back on sugar scared me," says Auerbach Berlin. "But within a week of starting the program and following the recipes, coffee with just a little stevia tasted great to me. I never would have enjoyed it that way before, but my taste buds really did change. Hooray for the small things in life!"

IT KEEPS YOU SATISFIED. Ever eaten a bag of chips or a handful of cookies only to find yourself opening the fridge or peeking into the pantry in search of your next snack within minutes? Well, that's probably because the snack you ate was processed and full of simple carbs and sugar or artificial sweeteners that spike hunger. When you're eating clean, whole foods, it's much easier to get the right mix of satiating fat, protein, and fiber that keeps hunger pangs—and your desire to nosh all day—in check. That's because whole foods aren't stripped of important hunger-staving nutrients, like fiber. High-fiber foods—like fruits, vegetables, and whole grains—require more chew time and take longer to digest, which can help you feel fuller longer. In addition to being high in fiber, fruits and vegetables have a higher water content, which adds to that feeling of fullness without packing a ton of calories.[4]

IT REVS YOUR METABOLISM. Starting at age 30, most people begin to lose about half a pound of lean muscle mass—the body's prime calorie-burning tissue and a key driver of your metabolism—each year. By the time you reach your late fifties, you could easily have lost nearly 15 pounds of the metabolically active tissue, a change that could cause you to gain nearly the same amount of body fat. However, research shows that, when combined with a little regular exercise, eating adequate protein throughout the day (about 20 to 30 grams at each meal) can help you rebuild muscle mass and ignite your metabolism.

That's why lean protein is such a vital component to a clean diet, and plays an important role in the Fit in 10 meal plan. Structuring your meals around whole, protein-packed foods like quinoa, beans and legumes, and organic dairy, meat, and poultry—rather than simple processed carbs—will help you give your body the nutrients it needs to power up your muscles' fat-burning potential.

Clean-Eating Guidelines

Ready to get started? Keep these simple principles in mind.

EAT WHOLE FOODS. This is the easiest way to stop eating dirty. A whole food hasn't been changed from its original form or been processed or refined in any way. Whole foods are nature's power foods, packed with the naturally occurring vitamins, minerals, and nutrients your body needs to feel and look its best. You'll find most whole foods along the perimeter of the grocery store or at your local farmers' market. Think fruits and veggies, organic meats and poultry, organic dairy, nuts and seeds, and whole grains.

While there are certainly some healthy and quick packaged foods that can make clean eating even easier, as a general rule—especially when you're pressed for time—anything that has been packaged is going to be processed to some extent. Some types of processing are less harmful than others and don't strip away the natural fiber and other good stuff, but most of the time the process winds up removing vital nutrients and adding sugar, fat, and chemicals. So by avoiding boxed and bagged foods most of the time, you'll easily get clean and lean.

READ FOOD LABELS. You won't be able to avoid packaged foods 100 percent of the time, nor should you. There are some great clean options out there, as long as you know how to spot them. That's why reading labels is vital, especially when you're just starting to purge the junk from your kitchen. Of course, if you find squinting at those tiny stats annoying, you're not alone. In fact, 75 percent of people barely give them a glance, and those that do read them tend to make the common mistake of only looking at the fat and calories of an item.[5] While you should keep those stats in mind; the nutritional value of a food isn't just about its caloric impact. Many low-cal, low-fat foods like diet soda and fat-free baked goods are loaded with chemicals or added sugar. Plus, as long as you're keeping servings in mind, healthy fats can make it easier to lose weight by helping you feel fuller longer.

Thankfully, the FDA is refreshing the design of the standard nutrition label, and by 2018 it will be easier to identify serving sizes and spot added sugars on any packaged goods.[6] Until then, it's time to start reading labels like a clean eater.

One of the first places to look is at the

SPOT ADDED SUGAR

No matter what it's called, added sugar means extra calories. If you find one of its many names listed on a food's label, consider leaving it on the shelf.

- Agave nectar
- Brown sugar
- Cane sugar
- Confectioner's sugar
- Corn syrup
- Dextrose
- Evaporated cane juice
- Fructose
- Fruit juice
- Fruit juice concentrates
- Galactose
- Glucose
- Granulated sugar
- High-fructose corn syrup
- Honey
- Invert sugar
- Lactose
- Maltose
- Maple syrup
- Molasses
- Raw sugar
- Sucrose
- Syrup
- Turbinado sugar

ingredient list. Ideally, you'll see a short list of whole ingredients, like apples, oats, or milk. If the list is long and full of complex words you don't recognize or could never buy solo—say, like the nasty preservative sodium benzoate[7]— it's best to leave that item on the shelf. Seeing chemicals, additives, or artificial sweeteners or colorings is a clear sign that it's not a clean food and it's probably something you don't want to put in your body.

Another thing to keep in mind when taking a careful look at the ingredient list: Substances are ordered by weight. So the closer an ingredient is to the top of the list, the more the product contains. If you see added sugar within the first few ingredients, that means that there is probably way more sugar in there than your body needs. So, Don't put it in your basket.

COOK AT HOME MORE OFTEN. Who doesn't enjoy a beautiful meal out with friends or family? Dining out is one of life's greatest pleasures and certainly not something you have to give up entirely when you eat clean. However, if you're like many people, restaurant meals and takeout have become the norm rather than an occasional treat. The average American adult buys nearly six meals or snacks from a restaurant each week and spends nearly half their food dollars on eating out, according to the United States Healthful Food Council (USHFC).[8] While you can certainly make smart choices when grabbing a meal at your favorite haunt (more and more restaurants are starting to cater toward the health-focused foodie), we all know that it's much harder to control the sourcing of ingredients or to know exactly how much sugar, salt, or fat is being added to your meals and drinks. Cooking at home allows you to know exactly what you're eating and makes it easier to control portion

sizes. Many restaurant meals clock in at more than 1,800 calories, the amount the USDA recommends sedentary women eat in a day.[9] Plus, with the right tips and tricks you'll find in the next few pages, cooking at home can be almost as convenient and just as delicious.

GO ORGANIC WHEN POSSIBLE—AT LEAST ON THE BIGGIES. Not every food that carries the certified organic label is ideal for your health or your waistline. There are plenty of snacks and sweets that are loaded with extra calories, fat, and sugar, so it's important to remember that organic ice cream is still ice cream (and should be an occasional treat, not a daily indulgence). However, when it comes to eating whole, real foods, opting for organic is a worthwhile investment in your health. Not only does buying organic help you avoid pesticides, as well as added hormones and antibiotics, many organic foods are also packed with more of the good stuff your body needs to look and feel its best.

When British researchers reviewed data from 263 published studies comparing the nutritional value of organic and conventional meat and milk, they found that the organic varieties contained around 50 percent more essential omega-3 fatty acids than conventionally produced products. That's a major incentive to buy organic, considering that omega-3s have been shown to help prevent heart disease and stroke, improve brain health, and reduce overall inflammation. The researchers also found that organic meats had lower concentra-

CLEAN UP YOUR COFFEE

If you can't get out the door without a cup (or two or three) of brain juice, there are quite a few reasons to keep up with that morning coffee habit. Coffee has been linked to a slew of stellar health benefits, including a lower risk of type 2 diabetes, heart disease, and cancer. Plus, research shows that drinking around 3 or 4 cups an hour before a workout increases your energy so you can go harder longer.[10] However, swirling in the wrong extras can dirty that cup quickly. One of the worst offenders: coffee creamer. Whether your go-to is French vanilla or hazelnut, these pseudo milks are often nothing more than water, sugar, oil, and chemicals. Plus, at about 30 calories per tablespoon,[11] trying to perk up your morning with a few heavy-handed pours

can pack on more than 12 pounds in a year.[14] And that's if you stick to only 2 cups a day.

While organic heavy cream or half-and-half is certainly cleaner than artificial creamers, it still adds calories (52 calories and 20 calories per tablespoon respectively). So if you're going to enjoy them daily, rein in how much you pour into each cup.

Lastly, sweeten up smarter. Instead of adding sugar or artificial sweeteners, try adding flavor with cleaner alternatives like cinnamon, vanilla extract, or unsweetened cocoa powder. Using naturally flavored coffee beans can also add a pleasant taste without the calories or chemicals. If you really need a touch of sweetness, opt for stevia.

---

tions of saturated fat, and that organic milk carried 40 percent more conjugated linoleic acid (a compound that may make it easier to stay at a healthy weight),[12] as well as higher concentrations of iron and vitamin E.[13] It makes sense when you consider that organic animals tend to eat healthier; their diets are mostly grass rather than grains, resulting in more nutrient-packed foods.

When it comes to fruits and veggies, organic is certainly best. The US Department of Agriculture's most recent testing in 2014 found widespread pesticide contamination on common produce. According to the Environ-

mental Working Group (EWG), at least one pesticide was found on nearly 75 percent of the samples tested, all of which were analyzed as typically eaten (which means they had been washed and, if applicable, peeled).[15] Gross, right? Thankfully, there are a few corners you can cut, as some produce is much cleaner than others. Check out the EWG's clean and dirty shopping guides on the following page.

TAILOR IT TO YOUR NEEDS. The idea that nutrition is a one-size-fits-all prescription is as outdated as cassette tapes. The way our bodies react to food is unique and can vary from person to person depending

SHOP SMART

While organic produce is best, you can buy conventional foods sometimes.

EWG's Clean 15 [16]	*EWG's Dirty Dozen* [17]
Okay to buy conventional	Better to go organic

1. Avocados	9. Papayas	1. Strawberries	7. Cherries
2. Corn	10. Kiwi	2. Apples	8. Spinach
3. Pineapples	11. Eggplant	3. Nectarines	9. Tomatoes
4. Cabbage	12. Honeydew	4. Peaches	10. Bell peppers
5. Sweet peas	13. Grapefruit	5. Celery	11. Cherry tomatoes
6. Onions	14. Cantaloupe	6. Grapes	12. Cucumbers
7. Asparagus	15. Cauliflower		
8. Mangoes			

on everything from genetics to the type of bacteria in our gut to how well our body responds to insulin (as mentioned previously, the hormone responsible for keeping our blood sugar at a healthy level). While we're arming you with these general clean-eating guidelines, only you know what's best for your body and if there are certain foods you—or someone in your family—can't eat. If there are foods you need to avoid, simply choose clean alternatives. That's what's great about clean eating. No matter what your diet limitations, you can make it work for you and your family.

BE SMART ABOUT PORTION SIZES. Simply making the switch from a highly processed diet to clean eating will improve your health and will help you lose weight and keep

it off. However, it is possible to have too much of a good thing. If you're eating clean and still not seeing the scale budge, it could be those almonds you're mindlessly noshing on at your desk every afternoon. After all, no matter how clean a food is, it still has calories, and you'll need to keep portion in mind. In general, if you're following the Fit in 10 toning plan and otherwise have a sedentary lifestyle, aim for roughly 1,400 calories a day. If your job keeps you moving, or you're adding in additional activity (like a morning run), aim for roughly 1,800 calories a day. MyFitnessPal is a great free app for tracking calories on the go. If you follow the Fit in 10 meal plan and recipes, you'll stay in a healthy calorie ballpark naturally.

DITCH ARTIFICIAL SWEETENERS. By now you've probably heard that diet soda, "light" yogurts, and artificial sweeteners (including aspartame, sucralose, saccharin, and acesulfame potassium) are no longer the diet darlings they once were. Those little blue and pink packets, along with any product that contains the chemical sweeteners, have been linked to everything from an increased risk of type 2 diabetes to weight gain to heightened cravings and can even negatively alter gut bacteria.[18] "I ate a fairly clean diet when starting the Fit in 10 plan, but I hadn't realized that my attempt to use diet soda as a 'treat' while my family enjoyed dessert was actually just making me crave something more sweet and triggering unnecessary snacking," says test panelist Linda Cohen. "Within a week of getting off the artificial sweeteners, I was very surprised I could get through the day without 'needing' dessert or something sweet to end my meal."

It Doesn't Have to Take a Lot of Time

When you first learn about clean eating, it's easy to assume that you will have to devote nearly all your waking hours to shopping, planning, or preparing meals. Compared to the drive-thru, it's true that it will require more time—but there are a lot of simple little tricks you can employ to make it as quick and easy as possible. Yes, you'll need to prepare the majority of your meals, but you certainly don't need to follow complex recipes or buy a long list of obscure ingredients. Clean eating can be as elaborate or a simple as you need it to be. There are plenty of busy nights when my version of clean eating is nothing more than a premade rotisserie chicken and salad that I pick up on the way home from work (and it's delicious, every time).

Still, if you're used to ordering in or eating out, making the commitment to eat clean can feel like a major adjustment. Luckily, there are a few ways to cut corners that can make a mega difference in your sanity and your ability to stick with clean eating, even on the busiest of days. Here are six ways to slash the amount of time it takes you to eat clean.

OUTSOURCE YOUR SHOPPING. If you live in an urban area, there's a good chance that you have access to a grocery delivery service. Companies such as AmazonFresh and Instacart will deliver groceries right to your door, often the same day and for a minimal delivery fee. If you've yet to experience it, it's worth a try—I've found it to be a game changer for those busy days when just the thought of going to the store feels overwhelming.

PAY FOR PREWASHED PRODUCE. Yes, it's much, much cheaper to wash and chop all of that spinach, kale, and broccoli yourself, but if you know that you're not going to get around to it this week—or you've watched countless heads of lettuce go bad due to laziness (been there, done that)—fork over the extra cash and be done

(continued on page 142)

THE FIT IN 10 PANTRY

Keep your kitchen stocked with these simple ingredients
and you'll be able to whip together healthy, clean meals in a flash.

Beans and Legumes

Chickpeas, lentils, black beans—whichever you prefer, these inexpensive protein- and fiber-packed veggies are excellent meal starters. If you buy them canned, rinse them in a colander before using to reduce the sodium.

Boxed Stock

Keep boxes of low-sodium organic vegetable or chicken stock on hand for quick soups or to add flavor to quinoa or brown rice (just cook them according to the package directions using stock instead of water). Use them in place of water or oil when cooking veggies.

Coconut Milk

Use this nondairy alternative for homemade dairy-free "ice cream" (just add it to your blender with some frozen fruit, a little vanilla extract, or unsweetened cocoa) or in coffee.

Canned Veggies

While most vegetables taste best fresh, a few—like artichoke hearts, hearts of palm, and olives—are quick and delicious straight out of the can. Pureed pumpkin is great for smoothies, soups, and baked goods.

Chia Seeds

Packed with fiber, omega-3s, and protein, these delicious, gelatinous little seeds make simple breakfast puddings or you can add them to smoothies.

Healthy Flours

Grain-free flours like almond flour, chickpea flour, and coconut flour are fantastic for gluten-free pancakes, baked goods, and "breaded" chicken. Or opt for whole wheat over white all-purpose flour.

Gelatin

Not only is this powder packed with protein (around 6 grams per tablespoon), the amino acids it contains are believed to help heal inflammation, ease achy joints, and improve skin and nail health. Use regular gelatin in homemade Jell-Os and gummies or add the tasteless hydrolysate variety to coffee, smoothies, or juice.[19]

Nuts and Nut Butters

Keep raw nuts on hands for simple snacks or crunchy additions to salads and enjoy natural nut butters with sliced apples or as a hearty boost to smoothies. People who eat tree nuts (think cashews, almonds, and walnuts) are less likely to be overweight or have metabolic syndrome, according to a *PLOS ONE* study.[20]

> When shopping for canned goods, opt for brands that come in BPA-free cans.

Oils

Every clean chef needs a few healthy fats on hand. My go-to for cooking is avocado oil (it's packed with heart-healthy monounsaturated fats), while I tend to use coconut oil for baking (it's also packed with healthy fat and adds a nice nutty flavor). I prefer to save extra-virgin olive oil for salads.

Protein Powder

Adding a scoop of protein powder to your breakfast or postworkout smoothie is often the fastest way to ensure you're getting enough of the metabolism-revving nutrient you need. If you're able to enjoy milk products, opt for an organic whey protein concentrate (which won't contain trace hormones or pesticides). Whey contains the essential amino acid leucine, which helps stimulate the muscle-rebuilding process after exercise, making it the best choice for muscle recovery and growth.[21] If you avoid dairy, consider pea protein isolate or hemp protein concentrate powders.

Quinoa

This versatile seed provides 8 grams of "complete" protein per cup, delivering all nine of the essential amino acids your body needs. Use it to create everything from breakfast cereals to savory meals and side dishes.

Seltzer/Sparkling Water

This bubbly, zero-calorie beverage is the best stand-in for soda and comes in a bunch of natural flavors. Make sure to check the ingredient list to ensure that you're buying an unsweetened version.

Unsweetened Cocoa Powder

If you love chocolate, this antioxidant-rich powder is a must. Add it to smoothies, yogurt, or even coffee for a clean fix.

Vinegar

The deliciously tart flavor of vinegar can add complexity to dishes, dressings, and marinades. Numerous studies have found that acetic acid, the main component in vinegar, may reduce the negative effects of a carb-heavy meal and help lower blood sugar.[22] Plus, thanks to its high concentration of resveratrol,[23] balsamic vinegar may help reduce the risk of heart disease.

Wild-Caught Tuna or Salmon

One of the most convenient sources of lean protein, these fish definitely deserve a spot in your pantry. Just be aware that they do contain traces of mercury. Follow the FDA's guidelines and limit your consumption to no more than 12 ounces a week.[24]

with it. If it weren't for bagged salad fixings, I would never eat the amount of greens that I do.

KEEP CLEAN STAPLES ON HAND. Even if you enjoy cooking, it's unrealistic to expect that you'll always cook everything from scratch. For those moments, it's vital to have a few clean items in the pantry that will help you throw together a quick meal (see page 140). And for those days when you just can't imagine cooking at all, you'll want to have a few clean packaged foods on hand.

ALWAYS AIM FOR LEFTOVERS. If you're already cooking dinner, why not make a little extra for tomorrow's lunch or dinner? By cooking in larger batches, you'll trim down the amount of time and effort you spend in the kitchen and ensure that you'll be set for the following day.

DO SOME PREP WORK. While this does take time and planning, identifying a few key ingredients you can make ahead for those super crazy days will ultimately save you a lot of stress and time when you need it most.

BE SMART ABOUT CLEANUP. You finally pop that casserole into the oven only to turn around to face messy countertops and an epic pile of dirty pots and pans. Delegating dish duty to your kids or partner (you cooked, after all) is one way to lessen the burden. A few others: Seek out simple, one-pot recipes that don't require heavy cleanup, and try to put away ingredients and wipe up spills as you go. In the end, it can save you quite a few precious minutes.

Let's Talk Food Prep

Social media is full of photos from people I like to think of as make-ahead mavens: extremely organized clean chefs who seemingly spend their entire weekend putting together beautifully prepared and carefully packaged meals for the week. While I admire and certainly encourage anyone who has the interest and time to devote to that level of commitment, I'm happy to say you don't have to sequester yourself in the kitchen for hours in order to make eating clean the rest of the week possible. There are plenty of super simple meals that take no more than 10 minutes of hands-on time (see the recipes starting on page 161), making it easy to whip up meals based on your mood or what you have in the fridge that day.

However, when your goal is to eat clean consistently, it can be super helpful to have a few key staples on hand, especially on groggy mornings, hectic evenings, or during those *hangry* (hunger + anger = hangry) moments when you're ready to shove just about any food in your face—no matter its nutrient density. Additionally, research shows that people who take time to prep meals eat healthier and lose more weight than those who don't plan ahead.

Of course, everyone and every family is unique and has their own likes and dislikes, so there isn't one magic list of foods you should prep ahead. The goal is to identify the healthy, clean staples that you have time to make on the weekend and that would make the task of putting together the clean meals and snacks you enjoy less daunting later in the week. You don't have to be wed to Sundays or the idea of prepping everything all at once, either; find a schedule that works for you and stay flexible.

Here are some great ideas to get you started. Then, my personal suggestion? Put on your favorite playlist or an interesting new podcast, and get prepping.

● **COOK YOUR FAVORITE CLEAN CARBS.** Quinoa and brown rice are the perfect bases for delicious, energizing breakfasts (page 172) and are ideal dinner accompaniments for any lean protein or stir-fry (pages 205 and 227). Unfortunately, their long cook times can make these hearty carbs tough to enjoy regularly, which is why I'll often take a few minutes at the end of the weekend to prep them for the week ahead. If you're an oatmeal fan, you can also do the same with steel-cut oats. They'll last in the fridge for up to a week and up to 3 months in the freezer. If you're eating for one, consider storing each serving separately to help with portion control. Be sure to cool completely before freezing in freezer bags. When reheating a frozen portion, remove the serving from the bag and place it in a microwave-safe container (no need to thaw). If you're using "the frozen quinoa or brown rice in a stir-fry, there's no need to reheat before tossing it in a

hot pan. Want to make your life even easier? All three of these hearty carbs can be made in a rice cooker, which means all you need to do is toss everything in, set the timer, and walk away. Depending on the size of the cooker, you can make anywhere from 6 to 20 cooked cups of yummy, fluffy, clean grains at a time. How's that for simple?

● **WASH AND CHOP PRODUCE.** Although I don't have time for it every week, I try to keep a rainbow of colorfully bagged fruits and veggies in the fridge: lettuce, kale, cucumbers, cauliflower, celery, red peppers, and whatever else I picked up at the market. I've found it to be one of the best ways to ensure I eat clean all week long. With salad, stir-fry, and smoothie ingredients ready to go, it takes only minutes to assemble just about any meal. All you need to do is add some lean protein, a little healthy fat, and you'll be well on your way to a delicious breakfast, lunch, or dinner. If I know I won't have time to prep—or I'm just not in the mood—I spend the extra money for prewashed salad greens, cauliflower "rice," and pre-chopped or frozen fruits and veggies. They're true lifesavers when you're short on time.

● **PREP CLEAN PROTEIN.** Eating adequate protein at regular intervals throughout the day is the key to maintaining and building lean muscle mass—and it's a lot easier to follow through on that goal when you have prepared options on hand (uncooked chicken breasts can't help you when you're standing in front of the fridge at 6 p.m. feeling starved). If you enjoy eggs, hard-boiling a dozen each week is a great start. A single egg has 6 grams of protein and comes in a handy, naturally biodegradable package, making it great for an on-the-go snack or lunch. If your go-to protein is poultry, consider baking, boiling, or grilling up a few extra chicken breasts or thighs. Having extras on hand allows you to easily top off a salad or slice the protein for salads, stir-fries, or lettuce wraps.

● **ROAST SOME VEGGIES.** What do asparagus, beets, sweet potatoes, peppers, onions, zucchini, squash, eggplant, broccoli, cauliflower, and Brussels sprouts all have in common? They're incredibly easy to roast and then enjoy throughout the week. All you need to do is roughly chop up your favorites or whatever vegetables you have on hand, toss them in a bowl with a little oil, salt, and garlic powder, and then spread your assortment evenly on a baking sheet (I'll often use two sheets, so the veggies don't get too crowded). Roast them in the oven at 425 degrees for about 20 minutes, tossing them once or twice to keep them from sticking to the pan or getting overly done in any one spot. Store them in an airtight container in the fridge for up to a week. Throw them into a salad, sandwich, or omelet; dip them in hummus; reheat them for a quick side dish; or blend them into a pureed soup—however you use them, you'll be glad to have them around.

● **BREW FRUIT-FLAVORED ICED TEA OR WATER.** Having a pitcher of something cold, refreshing, and a little fruity in your fridge can easily help you kick a soda habit or squelch an afternoon craving. Simply place your favorite flavor combination of fresh fruit, vegetables, and herbs in the bottom of a pitcher or jar, press them firmly with a muddler or spoon to release the juices, and then fill the container with water or unsweetened iced tea. Chill in the fridge for a few hours or overnight for the best flavor. A few great combos to try: cucumbers and mint; strawberries, lemon, and basil; and oranges and blueberries.

Time-Saving Kitchen Tools

Keeping these on hand will make cooking clean super simple—especially when life's at its craziest.

DEPENDABLE SLOW COOKER. My husband and I joke that our slow cooker is our "second wife." She stays home and makes dinner while we go to work and make money to pay the bills. All joking aside, while making a slow-cooker meal does take a little planning, coming home to roasted chicken or simmering chili feels amazing at the end of the day—especially when it only took you 10 minutes to toss in a few ingredients and go.

Lori Lowell

It was a June morning in 2016 when Lori Lowell reached her breaking point. She had just climbed into her car to make the 15-minute commute to her office, and Lori was *exhausted*. It wasn't just the long hours she put in at work. She'd managed a team of 10 employees for the past 4 years, and the fast-paced environment was taxing but perfect for her.

No, it was everything else. First, she was physically run down. She hadn't gotten a decent night's sleep in months due to back pain. She'd always struggled with her weight, but she'd never been this heavy before–190 pounds. It was too much for her 5'6" frame. Plus, the weight had settled around her belly, making it harder for her to do the gardening she enjoyed.

On top of feeling physically awful, her chest was tight with anxiety. Her younger sister, Donna, was battling brain cancer, her father-in-law was in the early stages of Alzheimer's, and she and her husband, Ken, had to get their kids through college.

Just then her phone rang. It was her neighbor Charlene. "I just sobbed on the phone to her," recalls Lori. "I felt so out of control. I knew I had to make a change."

Lori started walking each morning with Charlene–a 4-mile loop around their neighborhood. Then Lori's sister-in-law told her about the Fit in 10 program and everything clicked into

AGE:	**59**
POUNDS LOST:	**13**
INCHES LOST:	**19.25**

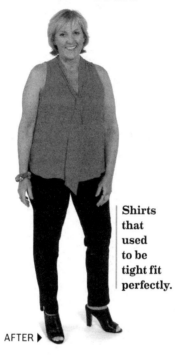

Shirts that used to be tight fit perfectly.

AFTER ▶

place. The clean eating and strength training appealed to her. She really liked that it wasn't a quick fix that she'd never be able to maintain.

Once she started following the meal plan and squeezing in the 10-minute routines, Lori was surprised by how quickly her energy and stress levels improved. "I felt proud that I was taking care of myself," she says. "I thought I'd be hungry, but my cravings were gone."

Within a month, Lori's back pain was gone, and clothes that had been tight were starting to loosen. By the end of the program, Lori felt years younger. On the weekends, when she was able to spend time in her garden, she didn't feel out of breath when she pushed the wheelbarrow or picked up lawn clippings. Getting dressed in the morning had gone from stressful to simple. "Before Fit in 10, I had a pair of jeans that were so tight that they were basically cutting me in half," she remembers. "Now, they're loose on me. It's an amazing feeling."

Why Lori Loves Fit in 10

IT'S EASY AND IT FIGHTS PAIN: "The program makes you feel good about what you can do and helps you build from there. My aches and pains have gone down 100 percent."

◀ BEFORE

1○-MINUTE LIFE CHANGER

Tune In to Taste

Most of us can easily remember a time when we were so busy or distracted that we sucked down a smoothie or inhaled a bag of chips without even tasting it. We've become so good at multitasking and being "connected" (to our smartphones, computers, TV) that we've lost our connection to food and the true enjoyment it can bring. So, what happens? Basically, we eat more and enjoy it less. How sad is that? In fact, research shows that we are also more likely to overeat and to feel less satisfied than if we'd taken a few moments to focus on the smell, texture, and taste of what we're putting into our mouths.[29] The good news: You can reboot the pleasure you get from food—and reduce your risk of bingeing—with this simple minute mindfulness technique.

1. Hold a morsel of food, such as a square of chocolate. What does it look and feel like?

2. Inhale deeply. Does its smell trigger a memory or feeling or make your mouth or stomach react?

3. Taste. How does it feel and taste on your tongue without chewing?

4. Bite. As it melts, how do the taste and texture change?

5. Swallow. How does it feel as it travels down your throat?

6. Reflect. How do you feel? You should be calmer and more satisfied after eating one tiny square than if you'd consumed the whole bar.

LESSON: It's often the quality of the eating experience, not the quantity of food, that increases pleasure.

KICKASS BLENDER. Smoothies are the ultimate clean fast food—unless you have to fight with a stubborn blender. Keep things quick and simple by investing in one that crushes ice and other hard ingredients. While going pro with a Blendtec or Vitamix will help you blend up silky-smooth smoothies for years to come, you don't have to lay down $500 or more if that's not in your budget. There are plenty of decent blenders that start in the neighborhood of $100 to $150. There's a certain pleasure that comes from pulverizing all of your icy or fibrous smoothie ingredients with just a flick of a switch.

CAST IRON DUTCH OVEN. This is, without a doubt, the pan I use most often. It's my go-to tool for creating one-pot dinners, especially on nights when I work late and just need to get something healthy on the table—and have zero desire to spend a lot of time cleaning up the kitchen. Normally, I'll start on the stovetop, searing whatever protein I'm using (often organic skinless, boneless chicken thighs) while the oven preheats. Then, I'll toss in a few chopped veggies (Brussels sprouts and sweet potatoes are regulars) and dust everything with some spices and a drizzle of olive oil. Within minutes, I'm popping it all into the oven to bake for a half hour or so (at about 425 degrees) while I go and do whatever needs doing. I don't mess around, and it turns out amazing each and every time. Bonus: leftovers for the next day.

VEGGIE SPIRALIZER. This awesome gadget turns zucchini, carrots, sweet potatoes, and other firm veggies into nutrient-packed, grain-free faux noodles. They're relatively inexpensive (most are under $40) and with just a few rotations of a hand crank, quickly create beautiful ribbons of veggies that can be used in cold "noodle" salads or tossed in a pan with a little garlic and olive oil for sautés or pseudo-pasta dishes.

IMMERSION BLENDER. While your main blender is a must for everyday smoothies, a hand blender is a fantastic little gadget for clean chefs who want to whip up pureed veggie soups or healthy side dishes quickly. (I love mine and bought it for no more than $20.) It's a must for some of my quick-and-clean faves, like mashed cauliflower or carrot-ginger soup.

SUPER-SHARP KNIFE. A dull knife can make chopping and prepping fruits and veggies painfully slow (not to mention dangerous). Even if you can't invest in an entire set, consider making a high-end chef's knife part of your clean cooking arsenal. When slicing through carrots, sweet potatoes, and tomatoes is like slicing through hot butter, you'll realize how ridiculously simple it is to whip up a quick stir-fry or salad. Knowing how quickly I can prep a meal has certainly helped me avoid giving in to takeout when I'm tired and my stomach is grumbling.

MANDOLINE SLICER. This tool makes the most complicated cutting jobs quick and simple. Use it to create translucently thin slices of almost any fruit or vegetable. It's great for baked potato or sweet potato chips; slices of zucchini or eggplant for veggie lasagna; a perfectly sliced tomato; or deliciously fine pieces of apple, pear, or orange for sandwiches, salads, or garnishes.

MICROPLANE ZESTER. This little gadget allows you to add vibrant flavor to any dish in seconds. Zest citrus skin, fresh ginger, or whole spices into salads, smoothies, sautés, marinades, or dressings for a fragrant, tasty boost.

SALAD SPINNER. If you're not going to buy prewashed lettuce, this ingenious device is a must for salad lovers. It allows you to wash and spin dry leafy greens (and fresh fruit!) in a matter of seconds.

FIT IN 10 FOODS TO ENJOY

Eat plenty of these foods to speed your weight loss and increase your health and energy.

Meat, Fish, and Eggs

All grass-fed meat, poultry, and seafood. Opt for organic grass-fed beef; free-range organic poultry and eggs; and line-caught fish. Canned fish is allowed.

Vegetables

Any fresh or frozen whole vegetables:

- Artichokes
- Asparagus
- Beets
- Broccoli
- Brussels sprouts
- Butternut squash
- Cabbage
- Cauliflower
- Celery
- Chard
- Collards
- Cucumber
- Eggplant
- Garlic
- Ginger
- Green beans
- Hearts of palm
- Jicama
- Kale
- Leeks
- Leafy greens
- Mushrooms
- Onions
- Parsnips
- Peppers
- Potatoes
- Pumpkin
- Radicchio
- Radishes
- Snow/snap peas
- Spaghetti squash
- Spinach
- Sweet potatoes/yams
- Tomatoes
- Turnips
- Zucchini

Fruit

Any fresh or frozen fruit (avoid canned fruit that contains added sugar), including these:

- Apple
- Apricot
- Avocado
- Banana
- Blueberry
- Cantaloupe
- Cherry
- Coconut
- Cranberry
- Grape
- Grapefruit
- Honeydew
- Kiwifruit
- Lemon
- Lime
- Nectarine
- Peach
- Pear
- Plum
- Raisins
- Olives
- Orange
- Strawberry
- Watermelon

Dairy

Opt for organic varieties with no added sugar or sweeteners.

- Milk
- Cheese
- Low-sodium cottage cheese
- Yogurt/kefir

Beverages

- Almond milk, unsweetened
- Coconut milk, unsweetened
- Coffee, espresso, unsweetened
- Hemp milk, unsweetened
- Kombucha
- Mineral water, water
- Seltzer water, unsweetened
- Tea, unsweetened

Spices and Herbs

All whole spices and herbs; avoid prepackaged mixes.

Condiments/Miscellaneous

- Broth, low sodium
- Cocoa powder, unsweetened
- Collagen, grass-fed
- Extracts (vanilla, lemon, almond, etc.)
- Nutritional brewer's yeast
- Mustard
- Protein powder, unsweetened (whey, egg white, hemp, or plant-based)
- Vinegars (apple cider, balsamic, red wine, etc.)

Nuts/Seeds

- Any raw whole nuts or seeds
- Unsweetened nut or seed butters
- Nut flours

Healthy Fats/Oils

- Avocado, avocado oil
- Coconut oil
- Grass-fed butter
- Ghee
- Olives and olive oil

Grains/Legumes

Limit to ½-cup serving a day. To slim faster, omit grains.

- Brown rice
- Beans (black, chickpeas, navy, pinto, etc.)
- Corn
- Lentils
- Millet
- Oats
- Quinoa
- Whole grain bread or tortillas
- Flours made from whole grains or beans

Sweeteners

Limit sweeteners to speed weight loss.

- Honey
- Maple syrup
- Monk fruit
- Stevia

FIT IN 10 FOODS TO AVOID

Avoid these foods on the Fit in 10 plan and revitalize your health and energy.

Processed/Refined Carbohydrates

Includes but is not limited to the following:

- Bagels
- Brownies
- Cake
- Candy
- Cereal
- Chips
- Cookies
- Cupcakes
- Energy/protein bars
- Pasta
- Pastries
- Pretzels
- Rice cakes
- White bread

Packaged/Processed Foods

Avoid fast food, frozen meals, and restaurant meals (see tips on page 136).

"Diet" or "Sugar-Free" Foods

See list of artificial sweeteners on page 135.

- Diet drinks (soda, iced tea)
- Gum

Beverages

- Alcohol
- Coffee "drinks" or shakes
- Juice
- Soda (regular and diet)

Condiments

- Store-bought ketchup
- Store-bought salad dressings
- Store-bought mayonnaise
- Coffee creamers

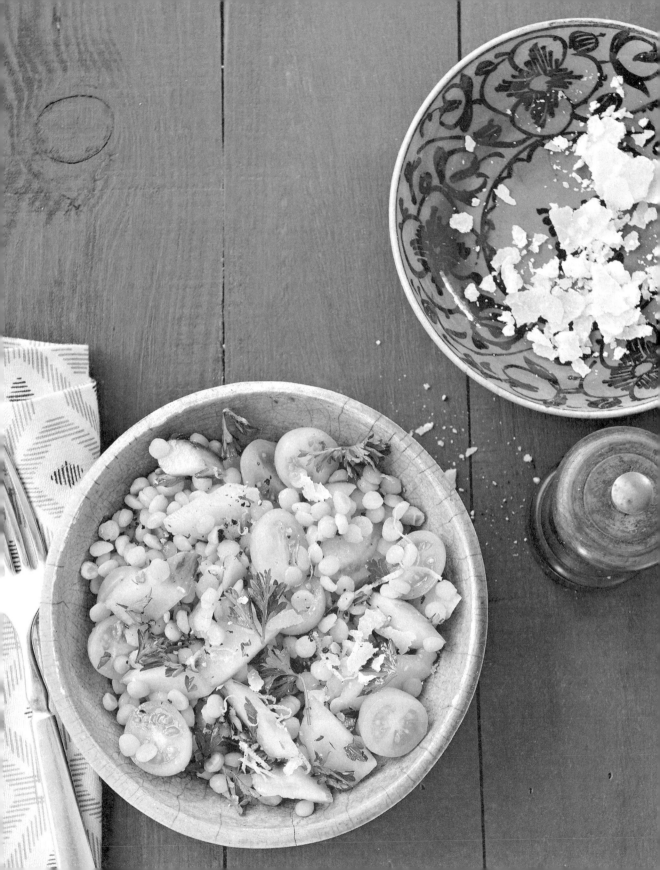

7

Your 10-Day Clean-Eating Jump Start

Many diet jump starts promise amazingly fast results–20 pounds in 21 days, for instance—and come with a long, miserable list of stringent rules. Food groups are often completely eliminated, calories are severely restricted (with some plans going as low as 800 calories a day), and intense daily exercise is mandatory. Not only are these types of programs completely miserable, but they're also not sustainable. When you're starving or following a long list of wacky guidelines that don't allow you to enjoy real food in the real world, it's incredibly difficult to stick with it long-term—which is why most people throw in the towel after a few days or

weeks and put any weight they lost back on very quickly.

The reason the Fit in 10 Clean-Eating Jump Start (see the chart on page 158) is so successful is because it's completely different. Unlike most detoxes, cleanses, and crazy diets, this plan isn't about restriction. It's about opening your eyes—and your stomach—to how delicious, enjoyable, and simple it can be to eat clean. Simply following the daily menus will ensure that you're meeting the optimal guidelines for safe, maintainable weight loss—about 1 to 3 pounds a week—while enjoying each and every bite. You'll never feel hungry, and you'll never feel like you can't eat like a normal person. Instead, you'll reboot your metabolism, gain new energy, and discover a bunch of great new recipes that you and your entire family will enjoy. Many of our test panelists found the plan so helpful and easy to follow that they repeated it multiple times.

"The Jump Start is a great way to become knowledgeable and comfortable with eating clean," says Lisa Berliner. "It showed me how simple it could be to make delicious food that's also healthy. I definitely wouldn't have had success without it."

Linda Cohen, who used to struggle with keeping portions in check, found it especially beneficial for breaking through a weight loss plateau. "Even though I was already eating relatively clean, I often ate more than I really needed," she says. "Once I began following the Jump Start, the pounds started falling off quickly."

Ready to take the stress and guesswork out of meal planning? Keep reading to get started.

How the Jump Start Works

The 10-Day Clean-Eating Jump Start carefully combines the Fit in 10 recipes that start on page 161 to ensure you're getting the perfect blend of metabolism-boosting lean protein while staying within a healthy calorie range for each day. Research shows that reducing calories while consuming adequate protein is the best way to safeguard your lean muscle mass while maximizing fat loss. When baby boomers exercised regularly and followed a moderate-calorie diet

(1,200 to 1,500 calories for women; 1,500 to 1,800 for men), while simultaneously increasing their protein intake to 1.5 g/kg of ideal body

10-MINUTE LIFE CHANGER
Prep Clean Snacks

We all know that there are days when life doesn't go as planned: Traffic jams, last-minute errands, long meetings, or a family emergency can throw your schedule into a tailspin. So for those moments when you're far from the fridge and your stomach is rumbling, it's essential to have a few clean snacks on hand. In fact, taking a few minutes each morning to prep your favorite on-the-go grub can help you avoid *hangret*—the regret you feel after eating junk food during a "hangry" moment.

So, what to bring? Sliced veggies, fruit, kale chips, organic beef or turkey jerky, and seeds and nuts all transport well. Freezable lunch bags (for information, go to www.packit.com) can keep perishable items—such as hard-cooked eggs or unsweetened Greek yogurt—cool for most of the day. Two of my favorite travel-friendly snacks: baby carrots and organic nut butter packs (like Justin's Classic Almond Butter).

Just be wary of processed treats that masquerade as health food, like sugar- or chemical-laced protein bars. Remember: If sugar or chemicals are on the ingredient list, it's not a whole food and it's probably not that clean.

weight—roughly 90 grams of protein if your ideal weight is 130 pounds—they lost nearly five times more weight than participants who exercised without changing their diets, according to a study published in the journal *The Physician and Sports Medicine*.[1] Even better: The calorie- and protein-conscious group gained more muscle, reduced their blood pressure, and dropped 2 inches from their waists.

Additionally, you'll score the right amount of healthy fat and good-for-you carbs to up your energy while minimizing cravings. Because you'll be eating consistently throughout the day, you'll keep your blood sugar levels more stable, which will reduce hunger and keep you satisfied. You can follow the 10-Day Clean-Eating Jump Start to kick-start your weight loss, or you can repeat it multiple times to keep the pounds peeling off.

How to Tailor the Plan to Your Dietary Needs

By now, we know that what's best for one person's body isn't always right for another's. With a few simple tweaks, however, the 10-Day Clean-Eating Jump Start plan can be modified to accommodate most dietary restrictions. Just be sure to use a free food journaling app like MyFitnessPal to ensure that the nutritional breakdown is similar to the original recipe.

IF YOU AVOID GLUTEN OR GRAINS. If you have celiac disease or gluten sensitivity or simply prefer to eat grain-free, you'll find numerous recipes to enjoy in the 10-Day Clean-Eating Jump Start and the Fit in 10 recipe section at the back of this book. (Look for recipes marked with this icon GF.) When a recipe does contain gluten or a grain, it can almost always be modified. Simply swap in your favorite Fit in 10 grain-free recipe or replace the grain with a different healthy carb, like quinoa, sweet potatoes, or your favorite vegetables.

IF YOU AVOID ANIMAL PROTEIN. If you choose to eat a vegetarian or pescatarian diet, you will find quite a few recipes that will work for your diet in the 10-Day Clean-Eating Jump Start and the Fit in 10 recipe section at the back of this book. (Look for recipes marked with this icon V.) If you eat a vegan diet, you can look for recipes with this icon VN, but you will have to make a few more modifications. Simply replace meat and poultry with plant-based alternatives such as tempeh, beans, or lentils. Choose your favorite dairy alternatives (such as almond or coconut milk and dairy-free yogurt) for smoothies, or simply use water and adjust the protein content by adding an organic plant-based protein powder that does not contain added sugar, chemical sweeteners, or fillers. Hummus, chickpeas, and seeds and nuts can often be swapped in for snacks that contain eggs or unsweetened yogurt.

IF YOU AVOID NUTS. Nuts are a great portable energy source, but there are plenty of options to enjoy if they don't work for your body or if a family member has an allergy and you

(continues on page 156)

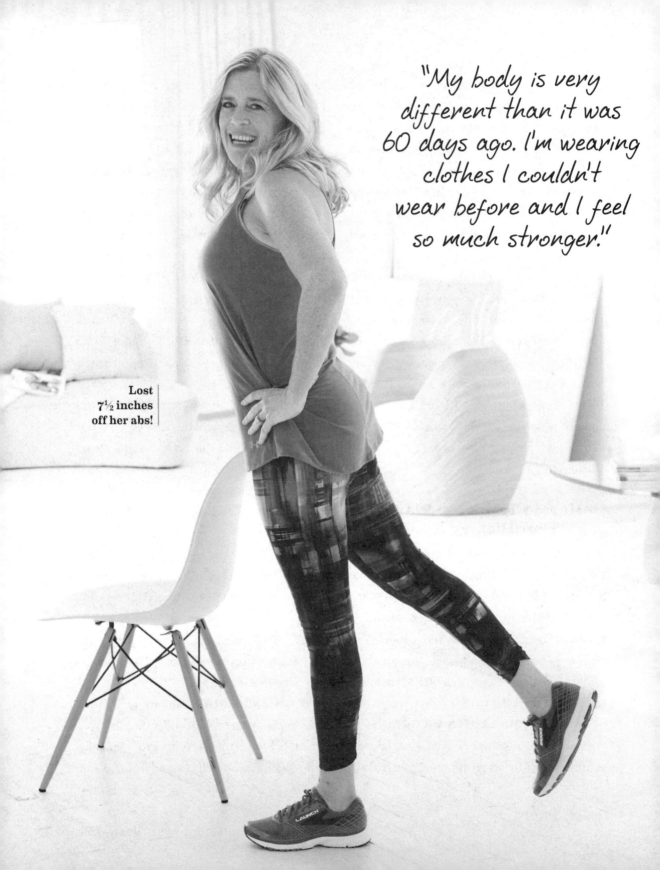

"My body is very different than it was 60 days ago. I'm wearing clothes I couldn't wear before and I feel so much stronger."

Lost 7½ inches off her abs!

Lisa Berliner

AGE:	**51**
POUNDS LOST:	**14**
INCHES LOST:	**19.75**

When getting dressed in the morning became a constant struggle, Lisa Berliner knew she needed to make a change. Over the last few years, she'd lost and gained 20 pounds multiple times with Weight Watchers and fad diets. She'd push herself to count carbs, points, and calories and then, sick of feeling so restricted, binge on high-calorie comfort foods, like pizza and mac-and-cheese. Working full-time as a realtor and juggling two teenage boys left her with little time to exercise. "I just wasn't feeling my best," she says. "I was dressing in tents; everything was an oversize tunic. I hated how stressed I felt every time I stood in front of my closet and tried to decide what to wear. But it wasn't just a fashion thing. Now that I'm over 50, I knew I really needed to start being healthy."

Craving a sustainable program that would show her exactly how to lose weight without losing her mind, Lisa decided to sign up for the *Fit in 10: Slim & Strong–for Life!* test panel after seeing a post for the program on Facebook.

At first, Lisa was nervous about the Fit in 10 meal plan–would she really like it? Would it really satisfy her? Would it feel like another diet? On the first day, she took a trip to the grocery store and bought the ingredients she needed for the 10-Day Clean-Eating Jump Start. "I felt a little intimidated, but once I got in the kitchen and started to make the meals, I realized how simple and delicious everything was. That's when I knew this program was going to be different from the ones I'd tried in the past." And Lisa wasn't the only one who enjoyed the Fit in 10 recipes. Her husband and kids loved them too. "As a mom, you don't want to be on such a special type of diet where you have to cook differently for your family," she says. "I loved that everyone in my house could eat the same foods. Our favorite meal quickly became the Hearty Lasagna (page 230). It was so delicious that my family started to request it."

Berliner also found it easy to fit the 10-minute workouts into her day. "Not only could I always find the time to do them, but the routines often gave me the energy to keep moving the rest of the day," she says.

By the end of the plan, Berliner was down 14 pounds, her clothes were fitting much better, and she couldn't believe the change she saw in her middle. "For the first time in as long as I can remember, my stomach is completely flat," she says. "And the rest of me feels stronger. I never would have thought in such a short period of time that I'd feel such strength in my upper body. The other day I carried my suitcase all the way up the stairs and through Grand Central Station–I never would have been able to do that if I hadn't started Fit in 10. It just makes me feel great."

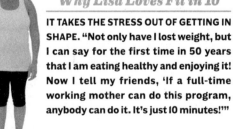

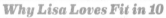

Why Lisa Loves Fit in 10

IT TAKES THE STRESS OUT OF GETTING IN SHAPE. "Not only have I lost weight, but I can say for the first time in 50 years that I am eating healthy and enjoying it! Now I tell my friends, 'If a full-time working mother can do this program, anybody can do it. It's just 10 minutes!'"

◀ BEFORE

prefer to keep them out of the house. If a recipe or snack calls for nut butter, opt for a seed butter, like sunflower or pepita (just be sure to pick a brand that doesn't contain added sugars), coconut butter, or try hummus or guacamole instead. You can replace whole nuts with

SIP TO SLIM DOWN

One of the easiest ways to up your energy, lift your mood, and make weight loss easier? Find a water bottle you love, take it with you everywhere, and refill it as often as possible. "Water serves many vital roles in the body, and it can be helpful for weight management in several ways," says registered dietician Brenda M. Davy, PhD, an associate professor of human nutrition, foods, and exercise at Virginia Tech Carilion School of Medicine and Research Institute. "First, it contains no calories, so it is a great substitution for high-calorie beverages such as fruit drinks or sodas. Second, drinking enough water can curb your appetite and reduce your calorie intake." In fact, when Dr. Davy and her research team had study participants drink 2 cups of water 20 to 30 minutes before each meal, the study participants ate 70 to 90 fewer calories than those who didn't chug a few glasses. That means you could trim up to 270 calories a day, a deficit that could result in a 28-pound weight loss in a single year.

Drinking enough water can also boost your metabolism, especially if you make your glass cold and frosty. When healthy men drank 500 ml of cold water they increased their metabolism by 30 percent within 30 to 40 minutes of chugging back that chilly H_2O, according to a study published in the *Journal of Clinical Endocrinology and Metabolism*. [2] The boost occurs because your body has to heat the icy liquid until it reaches body temperature, which requires energy and increases your calorie burn.[3]

Additionally, staying hydrated will increase your concentration, reduce your risk of headaches—and help you push harder when you pick up the weights. "If someone is not well hydrated and feeling fatigued, they may have trouble adhering to a daily exercise program," says Dr. Davy. "Physical performance can be impaired with even low levels of dehydration of about 1 to 2 percent."

Despite all of these amazing benefits, it can be tough to remember to keep your glass filled. "Most people need between 9 and 13 glasses of water a day, but the typical American drinks less than half that amount," says Dr. Davy.

That's why you should track your daily water intake in your journal. Many of our test panelists also found that drinking more water really improved the appearance of their skin. "Once I started getting 8 to 10 glasses a day, my face just looked brighter and healthier," says test panelist Anne Marie Russo. "It's an awesome side benefit." So swallow those excuses and make H_2O a priority.

your favorite seeds, olives, hard-cooked eggs, unsweetened yogurt, or any whole food that offers some lean protein and healthy fat.

IF YOU FOLLOW A LOW-SUGAR DIET While this plan is very low in added sugar, it does include natural sugars from whole foods (such as fruit and sweet potatoes). If you find that the smoothie recipes, for instance, have a little more natural sugar than you need, you can halve or replace the fruit with ice or leafy greens (kale or spinach are two of my favorites). You can also opt to swap a smoothie recipe for a Fit in 10 meal that doesn't contain fruit, such as Avocado Egg Boat with Smoked Salmon (page 166). The same goes for lunch and dinner. If a recipe listed has a higher carbohydrate count than you need, you can sub in starchy foods such as brown rice with an extra side of veggies or a little more lean protein.

WHAT IF I DON'T LIKE A RECIPE? If you don't like a recipe or snack in the 10-Day Clean-Eating Jump Start, or it doesn't work for your dietary limitations, you don't have to eat it. Instead, swap out the meal or snack for another in the same category. So, for example, if there is a breakfast you'd like to replace, swap it for another breakfast on the 10-Day Clean-Eating Jump Start or another Fit in 10 breakfast recipe that's similar in nutrition. This will ensure that your calories and nutrition remain within an optimal window for weight loss.

WHAT IF THERE'S A MEAL OR DAILY MENU I WANT TO REPEAT? If you find that you really love a particular meal and would like to enjoy it more often than it's listed, that's okay, too. There's absolutely nothing wrong with doubling down on the same meal if you really like it, especially if you have leftovers and want to eat them the following day. For instance, you may find that smoothies are best for your busy mornings, but an egg or protein-packed pancake recipe is perfect for the weekend. Or, if you're just cooking for one, and you make a dinner recipe that serves four, you could enjoy the leftovers throughout the week—which means you'll save even more time in the kitchen. So go ahead and use the Jump Start as an opportunity to discover which dishes you like and which are easiest for you to prepare.

Your 10-Day Clean-Eating Jump Start

Follow this daily guide to boost your energy, rev your metabolism, and speed weight loss.

Day	Breakfast	Snack	Lunch
1	Blueberry Muffin Parfait (page 184)	I small apple with I tablespoon almond butter	Mason Jar Mediterranean Salad (page 195)
2	Café Mocha Smoothie (page 165)	¾ cup plain fat-free Greek yogurt mixed with ¾ cup raspberries	Chicken and Bacon Pizza (page 191)
3	Pear-Ginger Smoothie (page 164)	Banana Peanut Butter "Ice Cream" Parfait (page 248)	Red Pepper Pesto Egg Pita (page 189)
4	Frittata Muffins (page 168)	¾ cup plain fat-free Greek yogurt mixed with ¾ cup raspberries	Rainbow Chard Chicken Wrap (page 203)
5	Banana-Almond Protein Smoothie (page 162)	Two large organic hard-cooked eggs	Chicken Salad Sandwich (page 192)
6	Bacon-Almond Pancakes (page 183)	¾ cup low-fat (1%), low-sodium cottage cheese mixed with ½ cup blueberries	Healthy Egg Salad (page 196)
7	Avocado Egg Boat with Smoked Salmon (page 166)	¾ cup plain fat-free Greek yogurt mixed with ½ cup grapes	Portobello Turkey Burger with Bruschetta (page 200)
8	Spinach Goat Cheese Egg Scramble (page 167)	I small apple with I tablespoon almond butter	Mason Jar Dijon Chicken and Chickpea Salad (page 186)
9	Cherry-Vanilla Smoothie (page 165)	Two large organic hard-cooked eggs	Mason Jar Citrus Chicken Salad (page 193)
10	Grilled Asparagus and Onion Hash with Fried Eggs (page 174)	¾ cup low-fat (1%), low-sodium cottage cheese mixed with ½ cup blueberries	3-Bean Salad with Sherry Vinaigrette (page 188)

Snack	Dinner	Nutrition Totals
Green Hummus and Veggies (page 246)	Chicken Stir-Fry (page 227)	**TOTAL NUTRITION:** 1,458 calories, 97 protein, 124 g carbs, 27 g fiber, 45 g sugar, 69 g fat, 14 g sat fat, 1,970 mg sodium
¼ cup roasted almonds (about 24 almonds)	Poached Salmon with Steamed Vegetables (page 225)	**TOTAL NUTRITION:** 1,445 calories, 121 g protein, 99 g carbs, 34 g fiber, 40 g sugar, 67 g fat, 17.5 g sat fat, 979 mg sodium
¾ cup low-fat (1%), low-sodium cottage cheese and ½ cup blueberries	Chicken Tacos with Tangy Guacamole (page 233)	**TOTAL NUTRITION:** 1,412 calories, 99 g protein, 112 g carbs, 46 g fiber, 52 g sugar, 53 g fat, 13 g sat fat, 1,563 mg sodium
Kale Chips (page 259)	Hearty Lasagna (page 230)	**TOTAL NUTRITION:** 1,372 calories, 123 g protein, 85 g carbs, 21 g fiber, 31 g sugar, 64 g fat, 21.5 g sat fat, 2,715 mg sodium
Spiced "Baked" Apple with Yogurt (page 252)	Pesto Chicken Bake (page 232)	**TOTAL NUTRITION:** 1,452 calories, 109 g protein, 119 g carbs, 22 g fiber, 54 g sugar, 63 g fat, 14 g sat fat, 1,573 mg sodium
¼ cup roasted almonds (about 24 almonds)	Spaghetti Squash Bolognese (page 234)	**TOTAL NUTRITION:** 1,474 calories, 95 g protein, 109 g carbs, 31 g fiber, 54 g sugar, 79 g fat, 14.5 g sat fat, 1,317 mg sodium
Cranberry Ginger Granola Bites (page 245)	Arugula Salad with Zucchini Ribbons (page 218)	**TOTAL NUTRITION:** 1,327 calories, 95 g protein, 92 g carbs, 29 g fiber, 40 g sugar, 71 g fat, 16.5 g sat fat, 1,325 mg sodium
Green Hummus and Veggies (page 246)	Speedy Fish Tacos (page 226)	**TOTAL NUTRITION:** 1,450 calories, 94 g protein, 121 g carbs, 28 g fiber, 34 g sugar, 72 g fat, 17.5 g sat fat, 2,665 mg sodium
Cranberry Ginger Granola Bites (page 245)	Almond-Encrusted Salmon with Greens (page 224)	**TOTAL NUTRITION:** 1,427 calories, 115 g protein, 102 g carbs, 17 g fiber, 72 g sugar, 65 g fat, 13.5 g sat fat, 1,044 mg sodium
1 small pear and ¼ cup walnuts	Broiled Steak and Smashed Potatoes (page 244)	**TOTAL NUTRITION:** 1,560 calories, 97 g protein, 120 g carbs, 35 g fiber, 45 g sugar, 80 g fat, 18 g sat fat, 1,998 mg sodium

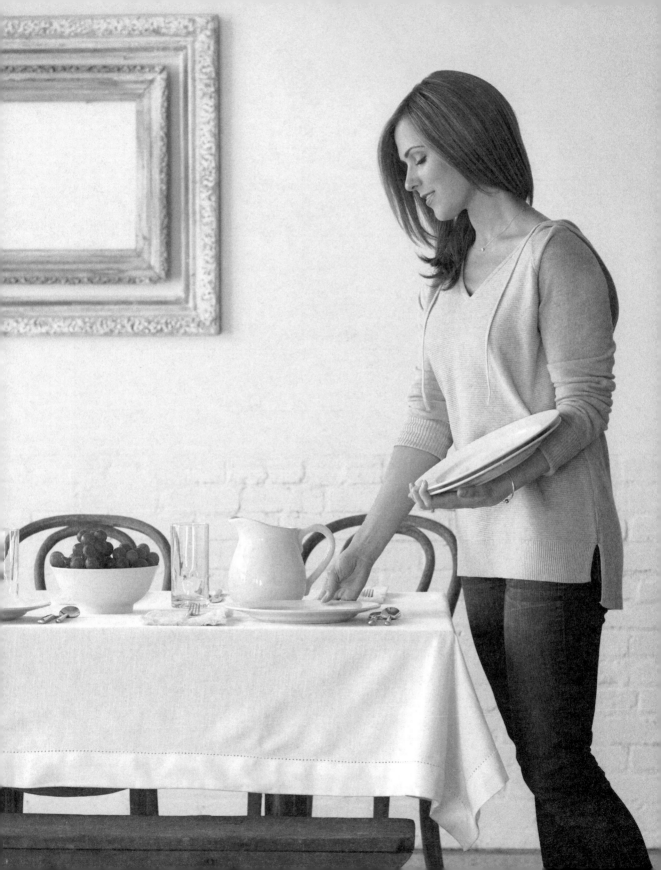

The Fit in 10 Recipes

Your taste buds are about to explode with happiness. That's because the 85 recipes in this chapter taste so amazing—and take so little time to make—that it's hard to believe they're actually good for you. In less time than it takes to order groceries online, you can easily throw together these fresh, wholesome 10-minute meals that are short on fuss, full of flavor, and perfectly balanced to help you get slim and strong for life.

This is not diet food—this is *real* food. There are refreshing smoothies and protein-packed breakfasts for your hectic mornings; clean, colorful, convenient lunches that travel easily; and mouthwatering dinners and desserts that feel like a reward to sit down to after a busy day. Knowing you can whip together wholesome dishes this good this fast makes eating for pleasure while revitalizing your health simply delicious.

And you won't be the only one looking forward to cake-like muffin parfaits dotted with fresh, juicy blueberries (page 184), hearty lasagna that puts a healthy spin on standard Italian (page 230), or pumpkin pie chia pudding (page 172). These are dishes your entire family will love. Check out the key below, and then flip through the following pages to find the recipes that will nourish your body and taste best.

- **FF** Family-friendly
- **GG** Great for a group
- **V** Vegetarian
- **VN** Vegan
- **GF** Grain-free
- **DF** Dairy-free
- **NF** Nut-free
- **10** 10 minutes or less
- **10+** 10 minutes or less hands-on time

Banana-Almond Protein Smoothie

PREP TIME: 2 MINUTES • COOK TIME: 1 MINUTE

This refreshing smoothie was a favorite among our test panelists. If you don't eat dairy, you can swap in a nondairy yogurt (coconut or almond) or just leave it out and add a little extra protein powder and water. Chia or flax seeds can be used in place of hemp seeds.

1½ tablespoons natural almond butter

2 teaspoons hulled hemp seeds

½ frozen banana, cut into chunks

¼ cup 2% plain Greek yogurt

¼ cup coconut water

2 tablespoons unsweetened vanilla whey protein powder

½ cup ice cubes

In a blender, combine the almond butter, hemp seeds, banana, yogurt, coconut water, protein powder, and ice. Blend until frothy, about 1 minute.

Serves 2

PER SERVING: 329 calories, 21 g protein, 26 g carbs, 5 g fiber, 14 g sugar, 18 g fat, 3 g saturated fat, 159 mg sodium

Pear-Ginger Smoothie

PREP TIME: 3 MINUTES • COOK TIME: 1 MINUTE

Energize your morning and wake up your taste buds with this nutrient-packed breakfast that disguises a full serving of greens behind the sweet and spicy flavors of pear and ginger. You can swap kale for spinach, if desired.

1 pear, cored and diced

2 cups baby spinach, rinsed

1½ cups unsweetened almond milk

1 scoop unsweetened vanilla whey protein powder

1½ teaspoons fresh lemon juice

½ teaspoon powdered ginger

½ teaspoon vanilla extract

¼ teaspoon ground cardamom or ⅛ teaspoon grated nutmeg

Blend the pear, spinach, almond milk, protein powder, lemon juice, ginger, vanilla, and cardamom or nutmeg until smooth and frothy, about 1 minute.

Serves 1

PER SERVING: 279 calories, 20 g protein, 40 g carbs, 9 g fiber, 19 g sugar, 6 g fat, 1 g saturated fat, 372 mg sodium

Café Mocha Smoothie

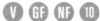

PREP TIME: 2 MINUTES • COOK TIME: 1 MINUTE

Dessert for breakfast is totally fine when it's full of satisfying protein and fiber, and this milkshake-like smoothie will quell your craving for ice cream in seconds. If you avoid dairy, you can easily sub in almond or coconut milk. If you want to reduce the natural sugars, experiment with using less banana and a little more ice.

¾ cup chilled brewed coffee

1 frozen banana, cut into chunks

½ cup whole milk

½ cup ice cubes

1 scoop unsweetened vanilla or chocolate whey protein powder

1 tablespoon unsweetened cocoa powder

In a blender, combine the coffee, banana, milk, ice, protein powder, and cocoa powder. Blend until frothy, about 1 minute.

Serves 1

PER SERVING: 285 calories, 23 g protein, 41 g carbs, 6 g fiber, 22 g sugar, 6 g fat, 3.5 g saturated fat, 102 mg sodium

Cherry-Vanilla Smoothie

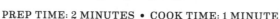

PREP TIME: 2 MINUTES • COOK TIME: 1 MINUTE

Even with only three ingredients, this fast and easy smoothie is simply delicious. If you avoid dairy, you can always replace it with unsweetened almond or coconut milk. Frozen blueberries are a great substitute if you don't have cherries. For an additional nutrient boost, toss in a handful of spinach or kale.

1¼ cups fat-free vanilla Greek yogurt

1 cup unsweetened pitted frozen cherries

½ cup ice water

In a blender, combine the yogurt, cherries, and water. Blend until frothy, about 1 minute.

Serves 1

PER SERVING: 297 calories, 28 g protein, 46 g carbs, 3 g fiber, 41 g sugar, 0 g fat, 0 g saturated fat, 113 mg sodium

Apple Pie Smoothie

  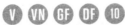

PREP TIME: 2 MINUTES • COOK TIME: 1 MINUTE

Satisfy your sweet tooth and your hunger with this icy treat that's full of mood-boosting omega-3s, plus satisfying protein and fiber. If you prefer, you can use 1% milk in place of almond milk.

1 cup unsweetened vanilla almond milk

½ cup ice cubes

1 apple, cored and chopped

1 scoop unsweetened vanilla protein powder

1 tablespoon walnuts

½ teaspoon cinnamon or apple pie spice

In a blender, combine the almond milk, ice, apple, protein powder, walnuts, and cinnamon or apple pie spice. Puree until smooth, about 1 minute.

Serves 1

PER SERVING: 277 calories, 19 g protein, 34 g carbs, 7 g fiber, 21 g sugar, 9 g fat, 1.5 g saturated fat, 223 mg sodium

Avocado Egg Boat with Smoked Salmon

   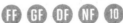

PREP TIME: 2 MINUTES • COOK TIME: 7 MINUTES

Rich and decadent, this simple breakfast is perfect for Sunday brunch—or any morning you want to feel special—and the mix of healthy fat, protein, and fiber will keep you full for hours. If you'd like, you could trade the raspberries for strawberries or blueberries.

½ avocado, peeled and pitted

1 large egg

2 ounces smoked salmon, thinly sliced

½ cup raspberries

Cut a sliver off the side of the avocado so it can lie flat in a pan. Crack the egg into the hole of the avocado, cover, and cook over low heat until the white is set and the yolk is cooked to your liking, about 5 minutes. Top with smoked salmon and serve with raspberries on the side.

Serves 1

PER SERVING: 331 calories, 19 g protein, 16 g carbs, 11 g fiber, 4 g sugar, 22 g fat, 4 g saturated fat, 523 mg sodium

Spinach Goat Cheese Egg Scramble

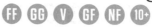

PREP TIME: 5 MINUTES • COOK TIME: 10 MINUTES

The few minutes it takes to assemble this elevated version of scrambled eggs is so worth it that many of our test panelists made it their go-to breakfast. Consider making a few batches at once for an even speedier on-the-go breakfast.

2 teaspoons olive oil, divided

1 scallion, sliced

1 small clove garlic, minced

2 cups baby spinach, rinsed

¼ teaspoon salt

⅛ teaspoon ground black pepper

2 large eggs, lightly beaten

1 ounce soft goat cheese, crumbled

1. In a large skillet, heat half the oil over medium heat. Add the scallion and garlic and cook, stirring frequently, until the scallion has softened, about 2 minutes.

2. Stir in the spinach, sprinkle with the salt and pepper, and continue cooking until the spinach has wilted and is heated through, 3 to 4 minutes. Transfer to a plate and cover to keep warm.

3. Add the remaining oil to the skillet. Add the eggs and with a rubber spatula or wooden spoon, start to pull them into the center of the skillet from the edges, allowing uncooked egg to flow into the skillet. When the eggs form soft curds, scatter the goat cheese on top and continue to cook until desired doneness, about 2 minutes. Top reserved spinach with eggs and serve.

Serves 1

PER SERVING: 332 calories, 20 g protein, I0 g carbs, 3 g fiber, I g sugar, 25 g fat, 8.5 g saturated fat, 927 mg sodium

Frittata Muffins

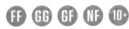

PREP TIME: 7 MINUTES • COOK TIME: 15 MINUTES

These egg-based "muffins" are so delicious you're going to want extra. Make a double batch and freeze the extra for busy mornings. Simply pop them in the microwave for 30 to 60 seconds to reheat.

1 tablespoon olive oil

2 cups loosely packed spinach (rinsed), arugula, or kale, chopped

4 slices Canadian bacon, diced

¼ small red onion, thinly sliced

4 large eggs

1 tablespoon whole milk

⅛ teaspoon kosher salt

⅛ teaspoon ground black pepper

1. Heat the oven to 400°F. Lightly mist 6 paper liners with nonaerosol cooking spray and place in a 6-cup muffin pan.

2. In a small skillet over medium heat, warm the oil. Cook the spinach, Canadian bacon, and onion, stirring, until the onion is soft and the spinach is wilted, about 4 minutes. Divide among the prepared muffin tins.

3. In a measuring cup, beat together the eggs, milk, salt, and pepper. Pour over the vegetables and bake until puffed and golden brown, about 10 minutes.

4. Let cool slightly before removing from the pan.

Serves 2

PER SERVING: 312 calories, 25 g protein, 4 g carbs, 1 g fiber, 1 g sugar, 21 g fat, 5.5 g saturated fat, 796 mg sodium

Sausage, Mushroom, and Pepper Scramble

FF GF DF NF 10

PREP TIME: 5 MINUTES • COOK TIME: 10 MINUTES

This one-pan meal makes cleanup as simple as the prep. If you have an extra minute, consider chopping a fresh plum tomato instead of using canned.

2 ounces loose
  pork sausage

½ cup sliced mushrooms

3 tablespoons finely
  chopped onion

2 tablespoons finely
  chopped green bell
  pepper

¼ cup drained petite
  diced canned tomatoes

2 eggs, beaten

½ teaspoon Cajun
  seasoning

1. In a medium nonstick skillet over medium heat, cook the sausage, mushrooms, onion, and bell pepper, breaking up the sausage with a wooden spoon, until the sausage is browned and the vegetables are tender, about 7 minutes. Stir in the tomatoes to warm through.

2. Push the vegetables and sausage to one side of the skillet and add the eggs to the empty side. Scramble until set, about 2 minutes. Sprinkle the seasoning over everything in the pan, stir everything together, and serve.

Serves 1

PER SERVING: 354 calories, 23 g protein, 9 g carbs, 2 g fiber, 4 g sugar, 25 g fat, 8 g saturated fat, 916 mg sodium

Baked Tomato and Egg Cups

FF **GG** **GF** **NF** **10**

PREP TIME: 5 MINUTES • **COOK TIME:** 10 MINUTES

This cheesy, grain-free breakfast is so delicious you won't even miss the toast. Use a sharp knife to halve the tomatoes and a small spoon to scoop out the seeds. If you find that your tomato halves are rolling around in the pan, you can take a thin slice off the bottom to create a flatter surface.

1 large plum tomato, halved and seeded

Kosher salt and ground black pepper

2 tablespoons chopped mixed herbs, such as basil, parsley, chives, oregano, or rosemary

2 large eggs

2 tablespoons grated Parmesan cheese

2 slices Canadian bacon

1. Heat the oven to 450°F. Place the tomato halves on a baking sheet and season with salt and pepper. Place I tablespoon of the herbs inside each half.

2. Crack the eggs and gently place in the cavity of each tomato. Season with salt and pepper and top with the cheese. Lay the bacon on the baking sheet.

3. Bake until the eggs are set and the bacon is crispy, 6 to 8 minutes. Serve the tomatoes with the bacon.

Serves 1

PER SERVING: 288 calories, 29 g protein, 5 g carbs, I g fiber, 2 g sugar, I6 g fat, 6 g saturated fat, 952 mg sodium

Savory Quinoa Porridge

FF GG V GF DF NF 10

PREP TIME: 3 MINUTES • **COOK TIME:** 6 MINUTES

This recipe makes great use of leftover quinoa. If you're already making it for dinner, toss in extra so you'll have ¾ cup on hand for breakfast.

¾ cup cooked quinoa

½ cup baby spinach, rinsed

½ cup drained and rinsed cannellini beans

1 tablespoon water

½ teaspoon olive oil or coconut oil

1 large egg

Salt and ground black pepper, to taste

1. In a large nonstick skillet over medium heat, combine the quinoa, spinach, beans, and water, stirring to combine. Cook until the spinach is wilted and the mixture is heated through, about 2 minutes.

2. Scoot the mixture to the side of the skillet and add the oil. Add the egg, season with salt and pepper, and cook until the white is set and the yolk is to your liking, about 3 minutes.

3. Scoop the quinoa mixture into a bowl and top with the egg.

Serves 1

PER SERVING: 345 calories, 20 g protein, 46 g carbs, 10 g fiber, 3 g sugar, 9 g fat, 2 g saturated fat, 511 mg sodium

Make-Ahead Pumpkin Pie Chia Pudding

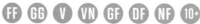 FF GG V VN GF DF NF 10+

PREP TIME: 5 MINUTES • **COOK TIME:** OVERNIGHT

Chia seeds are loaded with nutrients and, when soaked in the milk of your choice and touched with a bit of sweetener and spice, are transformed into a creamy pudding. Toss this together at night and wake up to a breakfast treat that will power you through your morning. You can use unsweetened almond milk in place of coconut milk if you prefer.

¼ cup pumpkin puree

¼ cup well-stirred canned coconut milk

1 scoop unsweetened vanilla protein powder

1 tablespoon chia seeds

½ teaspoon pumpkin pie spice

1. In a small bowl, whisk together the pumpkin puree, coconut milk, protein powder, chia seeds, and pumpkin pie spice. Alternatively, place the ingredients in a pint jar, seal, and shake vigorously to incorporate.

2. Cover the bowl and refrigerate overnight.

Serves 1

PER SERVING: 278 calories, 20 g protein, 17 g carbs, 7 g fiber, 4 g sugar, 17 g fat, 12 g saturated fat, 50 mg sodium

Banana-Cashew Oats

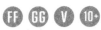

PREP TIME: 5 MINUTES • COOK TIME: 2 HOURS TO OVERNIGHT

This recipe is a perfect as a grab-and-go breakfast when made in a pint jar. Not a fan of cashews? Swap the cashew milk, cashew butter, and chopped cashews for their almond equivalents.

⅓ cup unsweetened cashew milk

½ cup 2% plain Greek yogurt

½ medium banana, mashed

2 teaspoons cashew butter

½ teaspoon almond extract

⅓ cup rolled oats

2 teaspoons chia seeds

½ teaspoon ground cinnamon

Pinch of kosher salt

2 teaspoons chopped cashews

1. In a cereal bowl or a pint jar, mix the milk, yogurt, banana, cashew butter, and almond extract until smooth.

2. Stir in the oats, chia seeds, cinnamon, and salt. Cover and refrigerate for at least 2 hours and up to overnight. Stir and serve cold, topped with the cashews.

Serves 1

PER SERVING: 417 calories, 20 g protein, 46 g carbs, 8 g fiber, 13 g sugar, 18 g fat, 3.5 g saturated fat, 239 mg sodium

Grilled Asparagus and Onion Hash with Fried Eggs

PREP TIME: 5 MINUTES • COOK TIME: 10 MINUTES

This warming breakfast packs a lot of tasty nutrients—including vitamins A, C, E, and K—onto one plate. You can use a cast iron skillet or your broiler to cook the asparagus and onion slices if you don't have a grill pan.

7 asparagus spears, tough ends removed

½ small onion, cut into ½-inch-thick slices

Kosher salt and ground black pepper

2 teaspoons olive oil

2 large eggs

3 tablespoons grated Parmesan cheese

1. Generously spray a grill pan with nonaerosol cooking spray and heat over medium-high heat for 1 minute. Add the asparagus and onion slices and grill, turning a few times, until tender, about 8 minutes. Transfer to a cutting board. Coarsely chop the onion and cut the asparagus into bite-size pieces. Toss together and season to taste with salt and pepper.

2. Meanwhile, in a medium nonstick skillet, warm the oil over medium heat. Crack the eggs into the skillet, season with salt and pepper, and cook until desired doneness, about 3 minutes.

3. Place the asparagus-onion hash on a plate, top with the eggs, and sprinkle with the cheese.

Serves 1

PER SERVING: 354 calories, 24 g protein, 9 g carbs, 3 g fiber, 4 g sugar, 25 g fat, 7.5 g saturated fat, 761 mg sodium

Soft-Boiled Eggs with Sweet Potato Soldiers

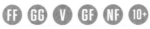

PREP TIME: 5 MINUTES • COOK TIME: 10 MINUTES

If you liked dippy eggs as a kid, you'll love this healthy twist on the childhood favorite. It subs in lightly crisped sweet potato "toast" for bread. Don't worry: Soft-boiling an egg is a lot easier than you think!

2 large eggs

4 slabs (¼ inch thick) sweet potato

Kosher salt and ground black pepper

2 tablespoons grated Cheddar cheese

1. Bring a 1-quart saucepan of water to a boil. Using a slotted spoon, gently lower the eggs into the water, reduce the heat to medium-low, cover, and cook for 4 minutes. Drain and immediately transfer to a large bowl of cold water.

2. Meanwhile, toast the sweet potato in a slot toaster until tender, 3 or 4 passes on medium-high. Alternatively, toast in a 400°F oven for about 10 minutes. While still hot, cut into ½-inch strips and sprinkle with salt, pepper, and cheese.

3. Place the eggs in egg cups and slice off the tops, or peel, cut in half, and lay on a plate. Sprinkle with salt and pepper to taste. Dip the sweet potato "soldiers" in the runny yolks and enjoy.

Serves 1

PER SERVING: 312 calories, 18 g protein, 27 g carbs, 4 g fiber, 6 g sugar, 14 g fat, 6 g saturated fat, 421 mg sodium

Overnight Oatmeal with Walnuts and Pears

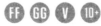

PREP TIME: 5 MINUTES • COOK TIME: OVERNIGHT PLUS 3 MINUTES

When you want something warm, satisfying, and slightly sweet, this recipe does the trick. Experiment with swapping in apple for the pear or using precooked quinoa in place of the oats.

⅔ cup fat-free milk

½ cup rolled oats

⅓ cup water

½ small pear, finely chopped

¼ cup fat-free vanilla Greek yogurt

¼ teaspoon ground cinnamon

1 tablespoon chopped walnuts

In a microwaveable bowl, combine the milk, oats, and water. Cover and refrigerate overnight. In the morning, microwave on high until heated through, stopping to stir every 30 seconds. Stir in the pear, yogurt, and cinnamon. Top with walnuts before serving.

Serves 1

PER SERVING: 352 calories, 20 g protein, 53 g carbs, 7 g fiber, 21 g sugar, 7 g fat, 0.5 g saturated fat, 112 mg sodium

Peachy Cottage Cheese Breakfast

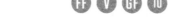

PREP TIME: 5 MINUTES • COOK TIME: 1 MINUTE

This recipe takes simple cottage cheese to a whole new level. If peaches aren't in season, thaw four slices of unsweetened frozen peaches and coarsely chop.

¾ cup low-fat cottage cheese

2 tablespoons roasted, salted cashews or almonds

½ peach, chopped

2 tablespoons toasted coconut flakes

In a small bowl, stir together the cottage cheese and cashews or almonds. Top with the peach and coconut and serve.

Serves 1

PER SERVING: 330 calories, 25 g protein, 20 g carbs, 3 g fiber, 12 g sugar, 17 g fat, 9 g saturated fat, 801 mg sodium

Power Pancakes with Fruit and Nuts

PREP TIME: 5 MINUTES • COOK TIME: 8 MINUTES

This recipe offers a refreshing, protein-packed take on pancakes. Share the extra serving or save the extra serving for tomorrow's breakfast.

4 large egg whites

1 large egg

¼ cup rolled oats

¼ cup low-fat
  cottage cheese

½ scoop unsweetened
  vanilla protein powder

2 teaspoons unsalted
  grass-fed butter

1 cup blueberries

1 apple, chopped

1 tablespoon chopped mint

2 teaspoons chopped
  walnuts

1. In a medium bowl, using a hand mixer, beat together the egg whites, whole egg, oats, cottage cheese, and protein powder.

2. In a medium nonstick skillet over medium heat, melt half the butter. Pour 3 circles of batter (scant ¼ cup each) into the skillet and cook until golden and no longer raw, 2 to 3 minutes per side. Repeat with the remaining butter and batter.

3. Toss together the blueberries, apple, mint, and walnuts. Serve the pancakes topped with the fruit and nut mix.

Serves 2

PER SERVING: 304 calories, 22 g protein, 33 g carbs, 5 g fiber, 19 g sugar, 10 g fat, 4 g saturated fat, 253 mg sodium

PB and J Oatmeal Cup

PREP TIME: 5 MINUTES • COOK TIME: 5 MINUTES

Warm and filling, this healthy twist on a childhood favorite is low in sugar, full of fiber, and big on taste. You can easily find peanut butter powder for sale online.

1 cup unsweetened almond milk

½ cup rolled oats

2 tablespoons peanut butter powder, such as PB Fit

¼ cup chopped strawberries and grapes

2 tablespoons 2% plain Greek yogurt

1 tablespoon finely chopped peanuts

1. In a microwaveable bowl or mug, combine the almond milk, oats, and peanut butter powder. Microwave on high until the oats are tender, 2½ to 3 minutes.

2. Stir in the strawberries, grapes, yogurt, and peanuts. Enjoy.

Serves 1

PER SERVING: 330 calories, 18 g protein, 40 g carbs, 9 g fiber, 6 g sugar, 12 g fat, 1 g saturated fat, 345 mg sodium

Simple Poached-Egg Avocado Toast

PREP TIME: 5 MINUTES • COOK TIME: 10 MINUTES

This breakfast has become a food blogger trend for good reason: It looks just as good as it tastes. Make sure your eggs are fresh for easier poaching.

2 large eggs

¼ avocado, mashed

1 slice sprouted whole grain bread, toasted

Kosher salt and ground black pepper

1 tablespoon thinly sliced chives or scallion

1. Bring a medium saucepan of water to a simmer over medium heat. With a slotted spoon, create a whirlpool in the water and crack the eggs into the water. Cook until the whites are firm but not hard, 3 to 5 minutes. Remove the eggs from the water with the slotted spoon to a plate.

2. Spread the avocado mash on the toast and cut in half. Top each half with a poached egg and season with salt and pepper. Sprinkle with the chives or scallion and enjoy!

Serves 1

PER SERVING: 305 calories, 18 g protein, 20 g carbs, 7 g fiber, 1 g sugar, 17 g fat, 4 g saturated fat, 461 mg sodium

Bacon-Almond Pancakes

PREP TIME: 3 MINUTES • COOK TIME: 7 MINUTES

When you can smell bacon and a pancake sizzling on the pan, it's a good morning. This recipe makes it possible in just 10 minutes and offers a grain-free way to start the day.

¼ cup almond meal

2 tablespoons coconut flour

2 tablespoons ground flaxseed

2 slices Canadian bacon, diced

2 large eggs

½ cup fat-free plain Greek yogurt, plus more if needed

2 teaspoons coconut oil

2 teaspoons maple syrup

Ground cinnamon

1. In a large bowl, combine the almond meal, coconut flour, and flaxseed. Mix in the bacon.

2. In a small bowl, combine the eggs and yogurt. Mix into the flour mixture until just combined. If the batter is too thick to drop from the spoon, add a bit more yogurt, a tablespoon at a time, until it's the proper consistency.

3. In a griddle or skillet over medium heat, heat the oil. Pour the batter in 4 circles onto the cooking surface, using ¼ cup per pancake. Cook 3 to 4 minutes, carefully turning once, or until lightly browned on both sides. Drizzle each serving with 1 teaspoon syrup and dust with cinnamon.

Serves 2

PER SERVING: 345 calories, 23 g protein, 17 g carbs, 6 g fiber, 8 g sugar, 22 g fat, 4 g saturated fat, 370 mg sodium

Blueberry Muffin Parfait

FF **V** **GF** **10**

PREP TIME: 2 MINUTES • COOK TIME: 5 MINUTES

This is a perfect on-the-go breakfast. Make the parfait in a jar, cap it, then take it with you. Our test panelists thought it tasted like cake!

- 2 tablespoons almond flour
- 1 tablespoon coconut flour
- 1 teaspoon ground flaxseed
- ½ teaspoon baking powder
- Pinch of ground cardamom or cinnamon
- Pinch of salt
- 1 large egg
- 1 tablespoon applesauce or mashed ripe banana
- 1 tablespoon fat-free milk
- 4 tablespoons fresh blueberries, divided
- ½ cup fat-free vanilla Greek yogurt, divided

1. Lightly grease a large microwaveable mug or ramekin. In a small bowl, combine the almond flour, coconut flour, flaxseed, baking powder, cardamom or cinnamon, and salt. Mix in the egg, applesauce or banana, and milk until fully incorporated. Stir in 2 tablespoons of the blueberries, then pour the mixture into the prepared mug.

2. Microwave on high until a toothpick inserted into the center comes out clean, 1 to 1½ minutes. Cool briefly until cool enough to handle.

3. Crumble half the muffin into the bottom of a small jar, bowl, or parfait glass. Top with half the yogurt. Repeat layers with the remaining muffin and yogurt. Top with the remaining 2 tablespoons blueberries and enjoy.

Serves 1

PER SERVING: 310 calories, 22 g protein, 25 g carbs, 6 g fiber, 16 g sugar, 14 g fat, 4 g saturated fat, 531 mg sodium

Mason Jar Dijon Chicken and Chickpea Salad

GF DF NF 10+

PREP TIME: 10 MINUTES • COOK TIME: 7 MINUTES

This recipe is a great make-ahead lunch that transports easily to the office. Prepping sliced veggies on the weekend makes putting it together even easier. Of course, you can always forgo the mason jar and toss together the ingredients in a mixing bowl.

1 tablespoon cider vinegar

1 tablespoon lemon juice

2 teaspoons olive oil

1 teaspoon Dijon mustard

$\frac{1}{8}$ teaspoon ground black pepper

$\frac{1}{8}$ teaspoon salt

$\frac{1}{2}$ cup sliced red or yellow bell peppers

$\frac{1}{2}$ cup shredded carrots

$\frac{1}{2}$ cup drained and rinsed no-salt-added canned chickpeas

3 ounces rotisserie skinless chicken breast, sliced

$\frac{1}{2}$ cup chopped tomatoes

1 cup mixed greens

1. To a 1-quart mason jar, add the vinegar, lemon juice, olive oil, mustard, black pepper, and salt. Screw on the lid and shake vigorously until combined.

2. In the mason jar, layer the salad ingredients in the following order: bell peppers, carrots, chickpeas, chicken, tomatoes, mixed greens. Replace the lid and refrigerate until ready to take.

3. To eat, shake the jar into a bowl or onto a plate; that should be enough to coat the salad with the dressing. If not, gently toss with a fork.

Serves 1

PER SERVING: 390 calories, 28 g protein, 40 g carbs, 10 g fiber, 10 g sugar, 13 g fat, 2 g saturated fat, 600 mg sodium

Mason Jar Veggie Tuna Salad

GF OF NF 10+

PREP TIME: 10 MINUTES • COOK TIME: 7 MINUTES

This savory salad is a delicious way to get your midday protein and veggie fix. If you'd like to keep this plant-based, replace the tuna with chickpeas.

2 tablespoons Dijon mustard

2 teaspoons olive oil

¼ cup chopped celery

½ cup chopped green beans

1 cup snap peas

4 ounces unsalted chunk light water-packed tuna

10 large black olives, sliced

½ cup halved grape tomatoes

2 cups mixed baby greens

1. To a 1-quart mason jar, add the mustard and olive oil. Screw on the lid and shake vigorously.

2. In the mason jar, layer the salad ingredients in the following order: celery, green beans, snap peas, tuna, olives, tomatoes, and mixed greens. Replace the lid and refrigerate until ready to take.

3. To eat, shake the jar into a bowl or onto a plate; that should be enough to coat the salad with the dressing. If not, gently toss with a fork.

Serves 1

PER SERVING: 372 calories, 36 g protein, 24 g carbs, 10 g fiber, 9 g sugar, 15 g fat, 2 g saturated fat, 823 mg sodium

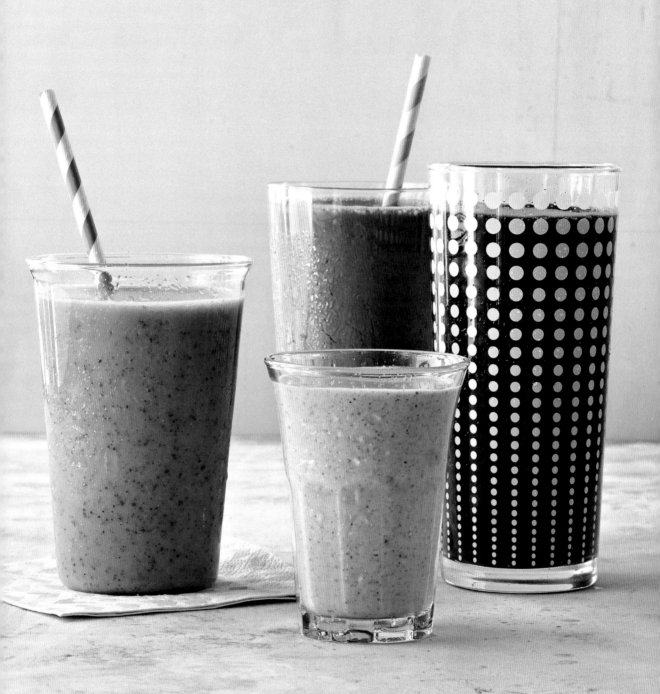

From left to right: Pear-Ginger Smoothie (page 163), Banana-Almond Protein Smoothie (page 162), Cherry-Vanilla Smoothie (page 164), and Café Mocha Smoothie (page 164).

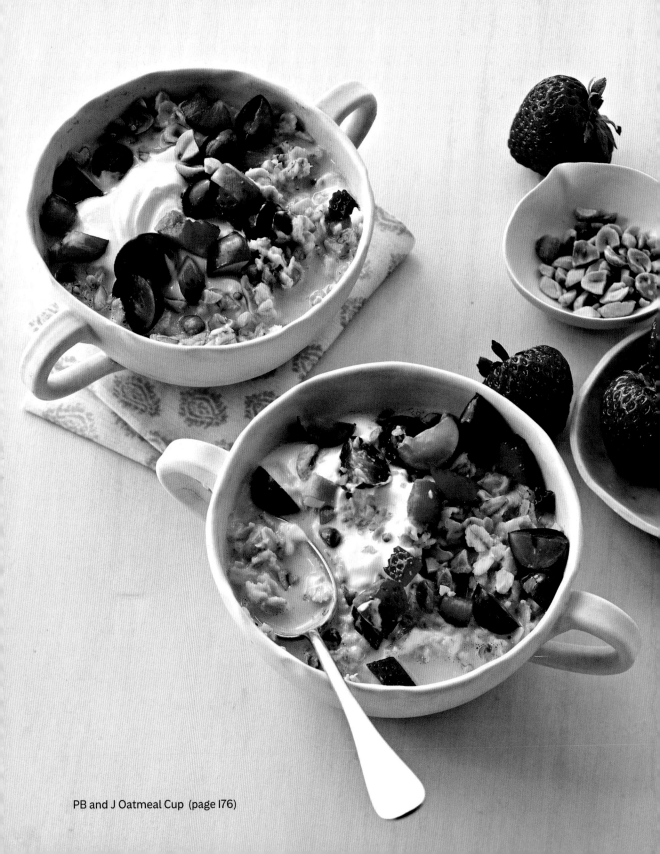

PB and J Oatmeal Cup (page 176)

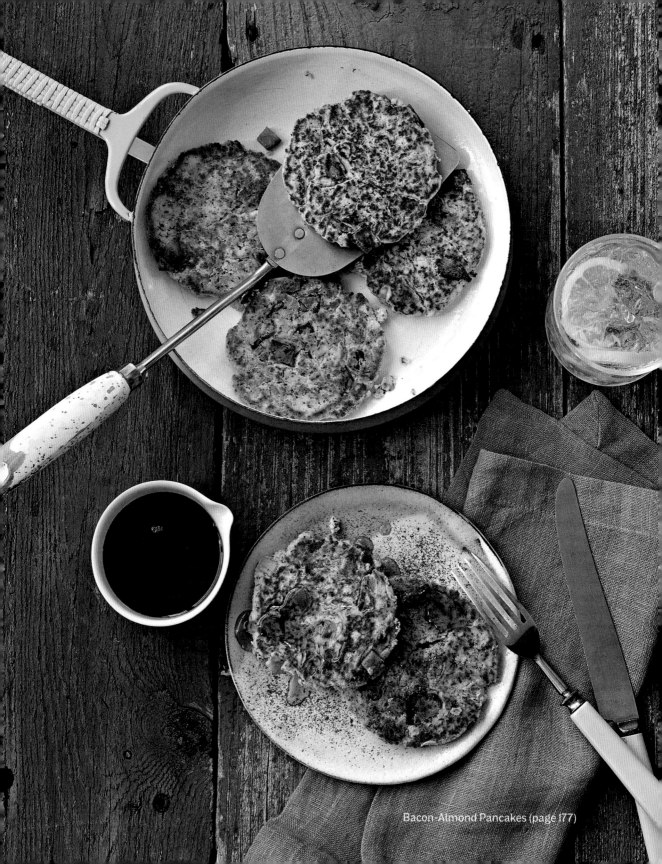

Bacon-Almond Pancakes (page 177)

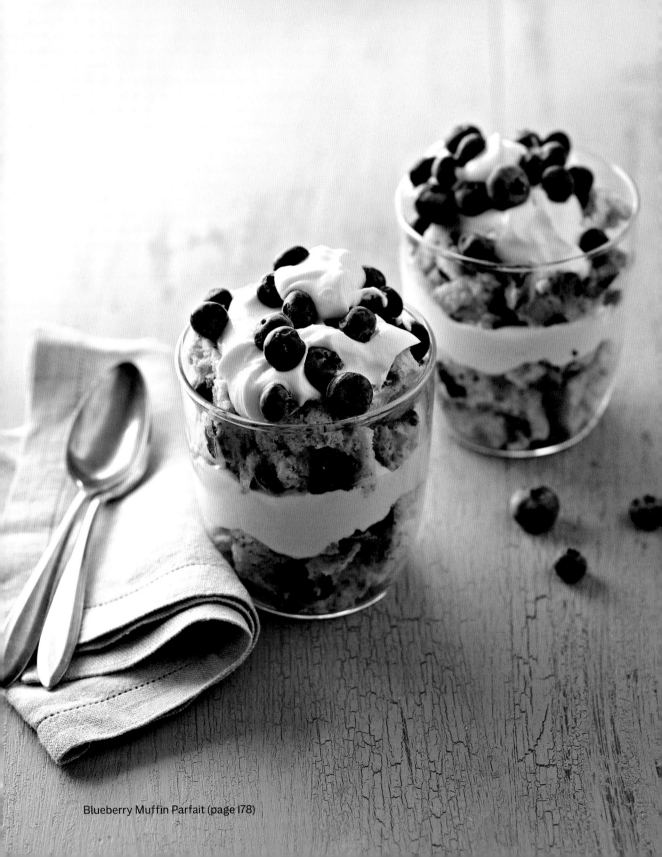

Blueberry Muffin Parfait (page 178)

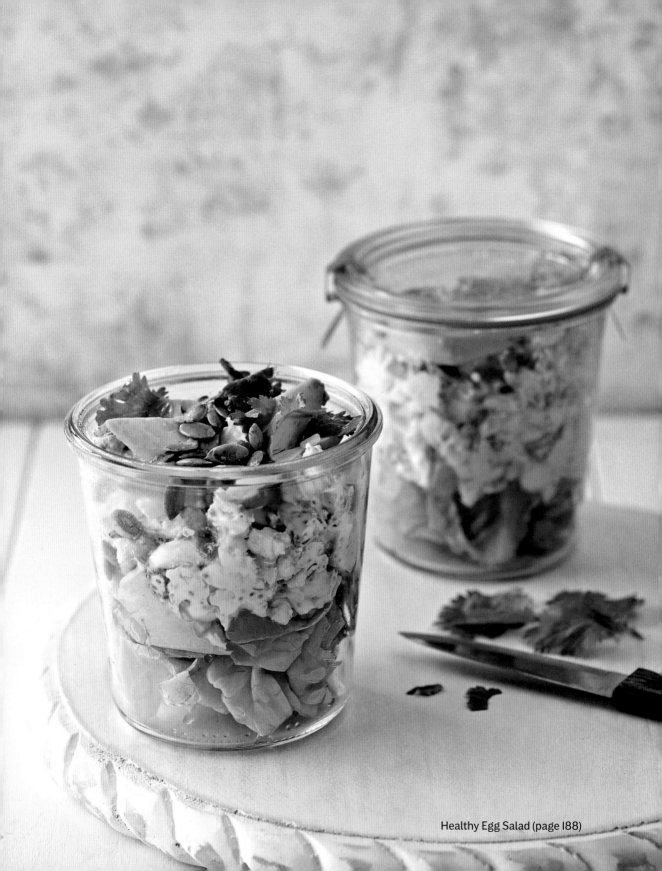

Healthy Egg Salad (page 188)

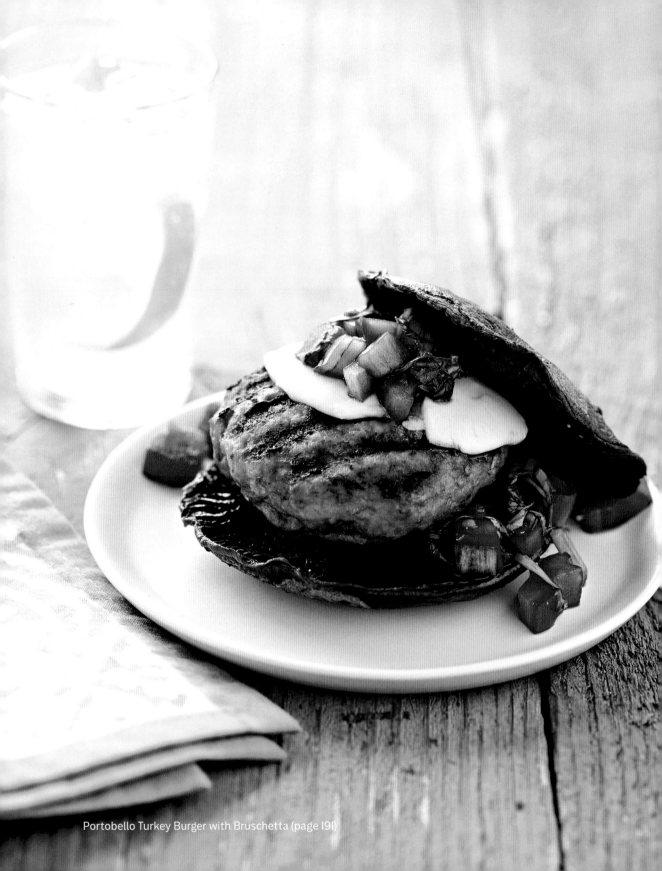

Portobello Turkey Burger with Bruschetta (page 191)

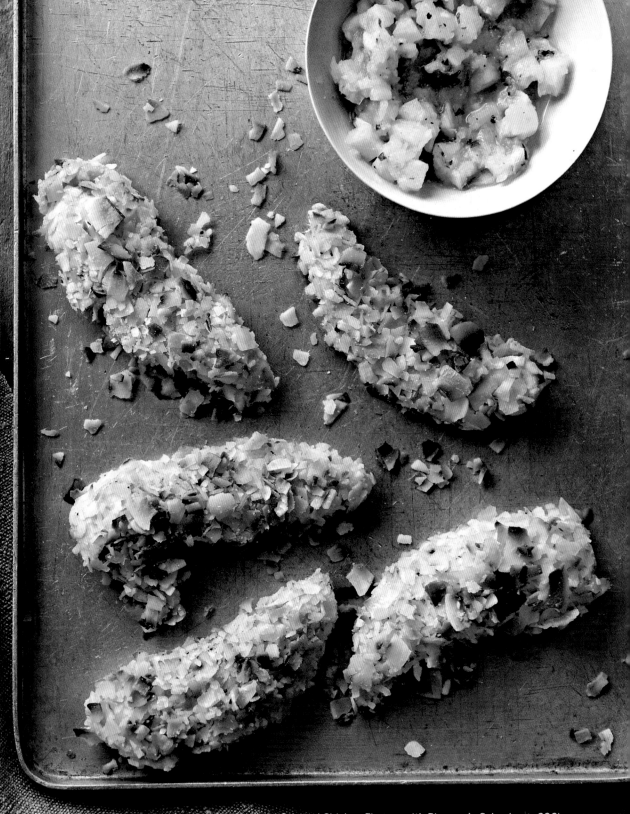

Coconut-Crusted Chicken Fingers with Pineapple Salsa (page 200)

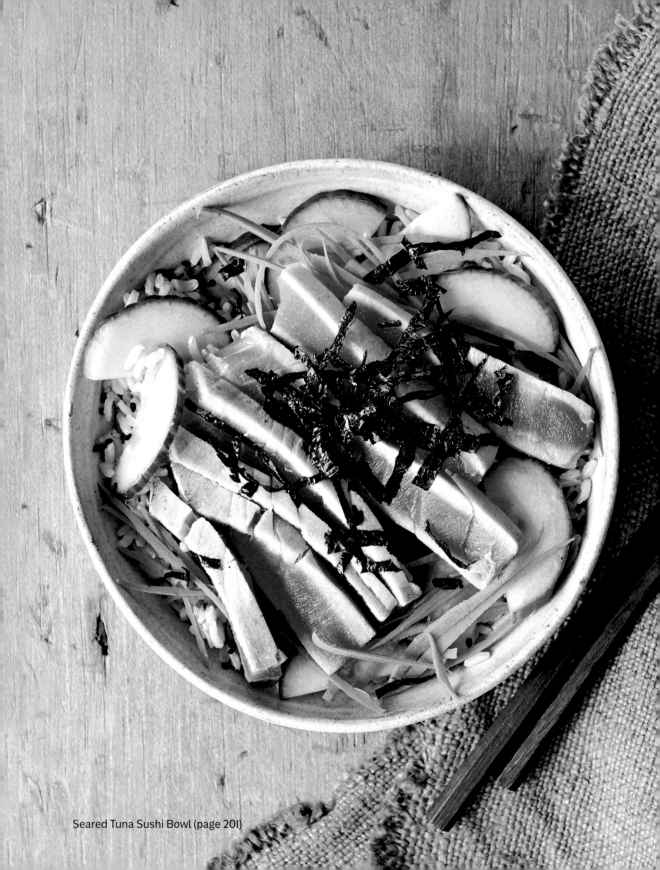

Seared Tuna Sushi Bowl (page 201)

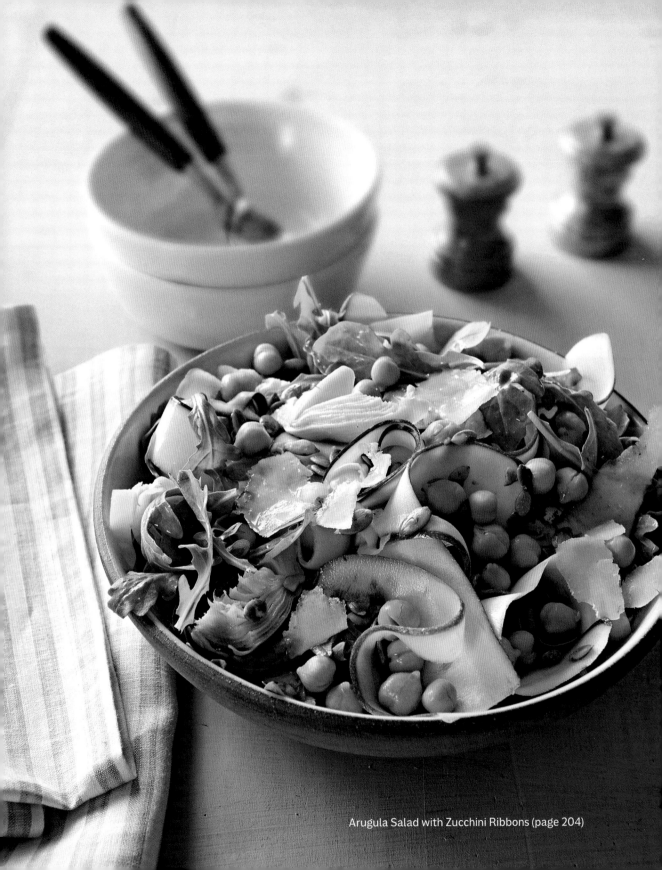

Arugula Salad with Zucchini Ribbons (page 204)

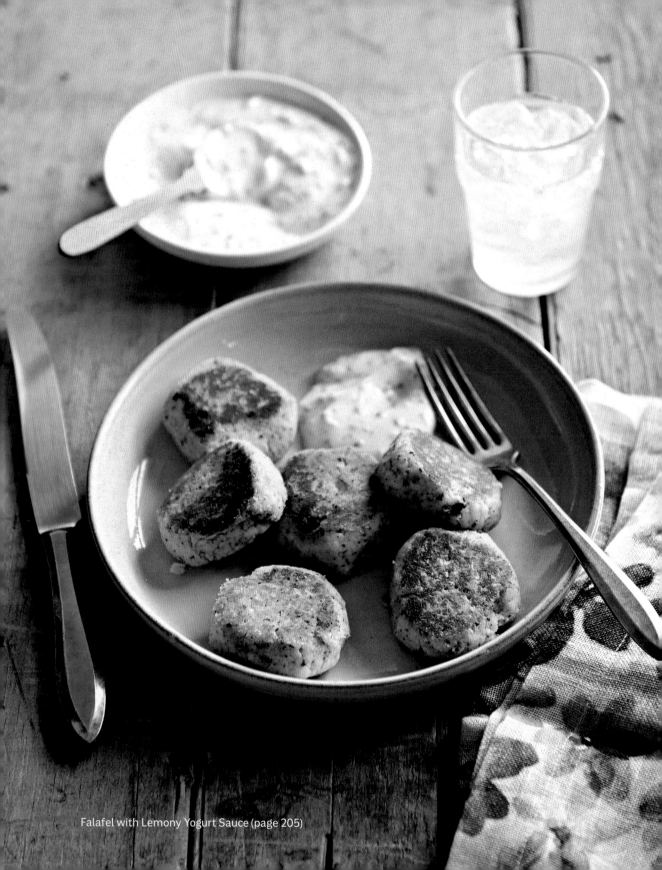

Falafel with Lemony Yogurt Sauce (page 205)

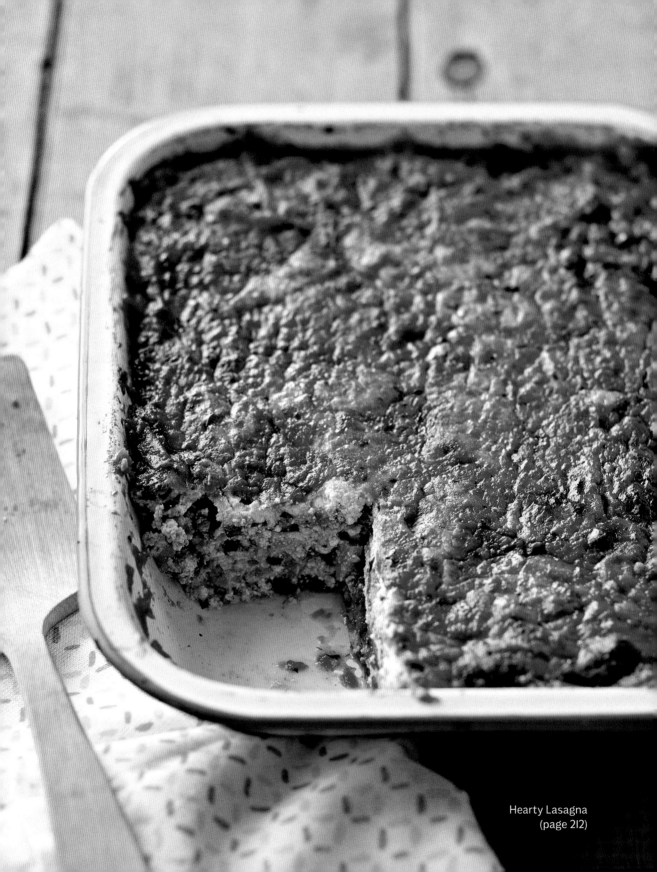

Hearty Lasagna
(page 212)

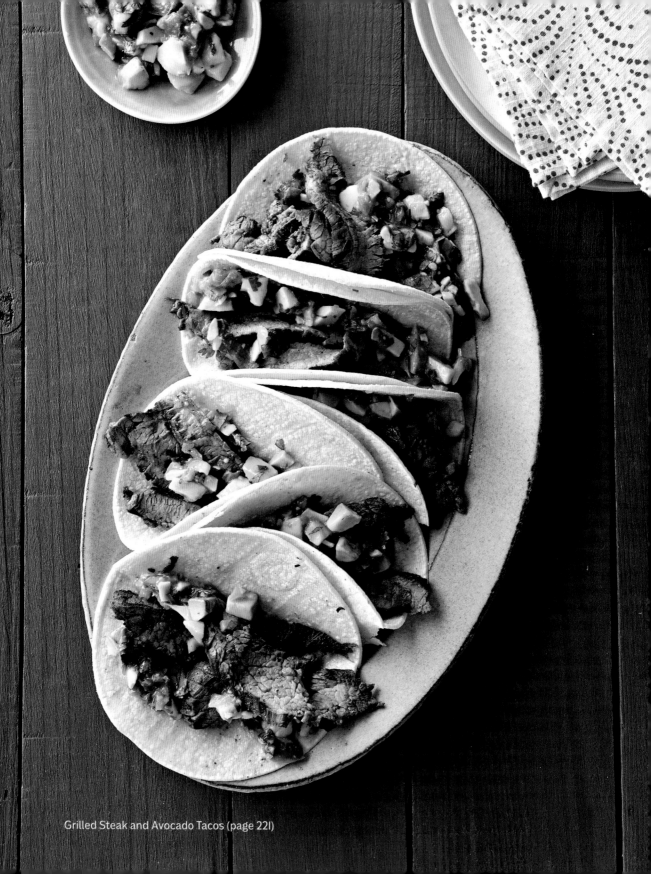

Grilled Steak and Avocado Tacos (page 221)

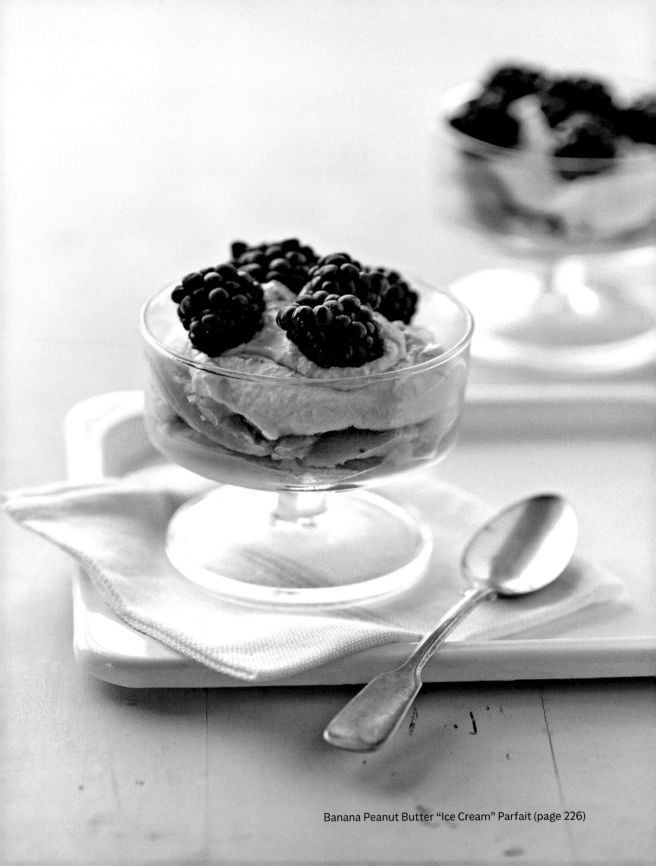

Banana Peanut Butter "Ice Cream" Parfait (page 226)

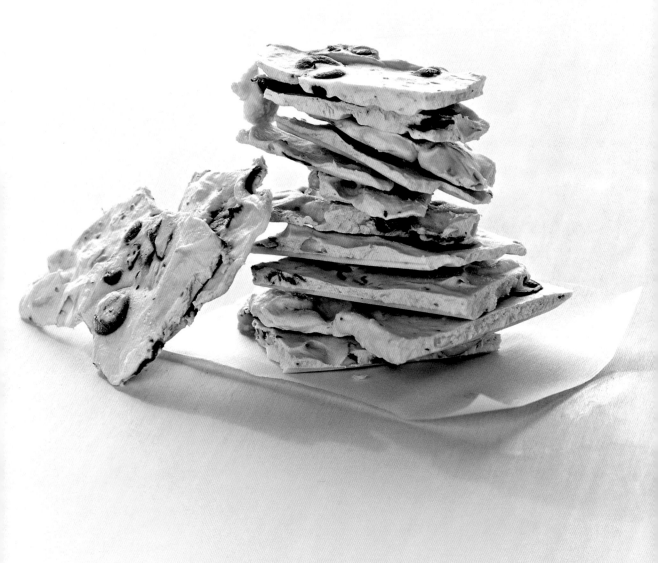

Blueberry-Hazelnut Yogurt Bark (page 230)

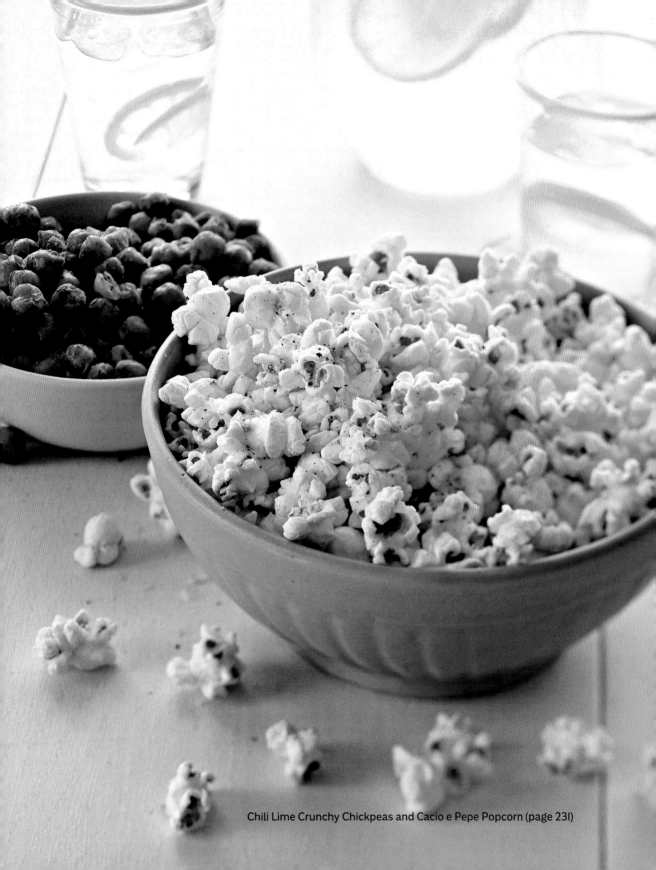

Chili Lime Crunchy Chickpeas and Cacio e Pepe Popcorn (page 231)

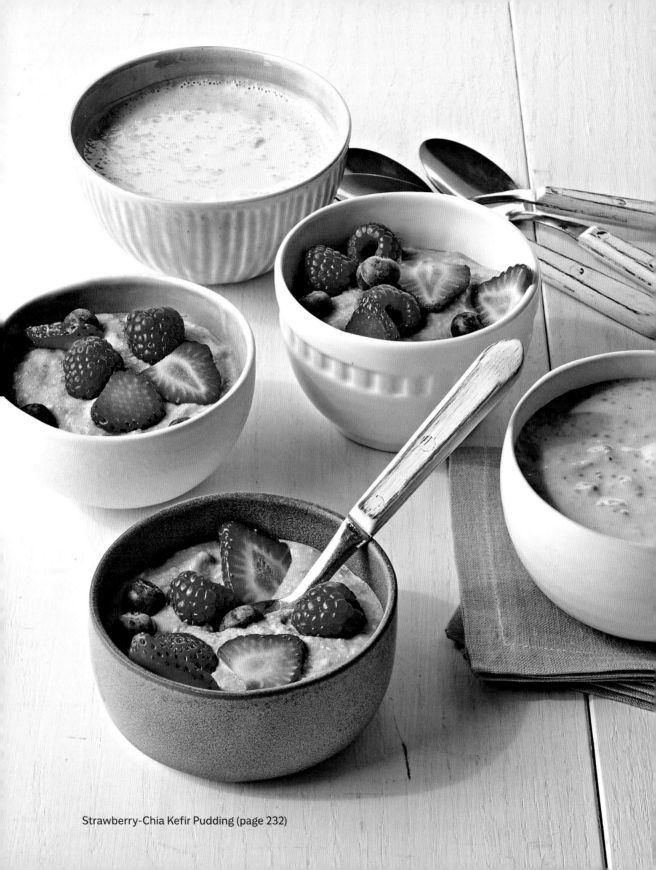

Strawberry-Chia Kefir Pudding (page 232)

3-Bean Salad with Sherry Vinaigrette

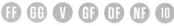

PREP TIME: 5 MINUTES • COOK TIME: 5 MINUTES

This hearty recipe can be made ahead, easily doubled, and kept in the fridge for quick meals throughout the week. If you avoid eggs, substitute a few slices of avocado.

½ cup halved fresh green beans

2 tablespoons water

2 tablespoons minced red onion

2 tablespoons sherry vinegar

1 tablespoon chopped parsley

½ teaspoon ground mustard powder or country Dijon mustard

¼ teaspoon ground black pepper

Pinch of salt

1 tablespoon olive oil

½ cup drained and rinsed canned lentils

½ cup drained and rinsed canned chickpeas

1 hard-cooked egg, chopped

1. In a microwaveable dish, combine the green beans and water. Cover and microwave on high until crisp-tender, about 2 minutes.

2. In a medium bowl, whisk together the onion, vinegar, parsley, mustard, pepper, and salt. Whisk in the oil. Toss in the lentils, chickpeas, and cooked green beans, coating with the vinaigrette. Serve topped with the egg.

Serves 1

PER SERVING: 446 calories, 22 g protein, 40 g carb, 17 g fiber, 6 g sugar, 22 g fat, 4 g saturated fat, 697 mg sodium

Red Pepper Pesto Egg Pita

PREP TIME: 4 MINUTES • COOK TIME: 8 MINUTES

Warm and satisfying, this recipe fills you up without weighing you down. The peppers and pesto add a boost of healthy antioxidants and flavor.

3 tablespoons reduced-fat ricotta cheese

1 teaspoon jarred roasted garlic

1 whole wheat pita

2 tablespoons chopped jarred roasted red peppers

1 tablespoon premade pesto

1 large egg

3 tablespoons grated reduced-fat mozzarella cheese

Pinch of ground black pepper

1. Heat the oven to 375°F.

2. In a small bowl, stir together the ricotta and garlic, blending well.

3. Place the pita on a baking sheet and spread the ricotta mixture on the pita. Arrange the peppers and dollop the pesto around the edges to contain the egg. Crack the egg into the center of the pita, top with the mozzarella, and season with the black pepper. Bake until the cheese is melted and the pita is crisp, about 6 minutes. Cut into wedges and serve.

Serves 1

PER SERVING: 386 calories, 23 g protein, 31 g carbs, 4 g fiber, 4 g sugar, 18 g fat, 7 g saturated fat, 621 mg sodium

Chicken and Bacon Pizza

PREP TIME: 5 MINUTES • COOK TIME: 12 MINUTES

This simple recipe satisfies your pizza craving and keeps you satisfied with hunger-staving protein and fiber. You can always trade the whole wheat tortilla for a gluten-free option.

½ teaspoon olive oil

½ teaspoon minced garlic

1 cup fresh baby spinach, rinsed

1 low-carb whole wheat tortilla (8-inch diameter) (We like La Tortilla Factory's organic non-GMO tortillas.)

1 tablespoon grated Parmesan cheese

2 ounces (⅓ cup) cooked chicken breast (from a rotisserie chicken), shredded

1 slice low-sodium turkey bacon, cooked and crumbled

1 ounce (¼ cup) shredded mozzarella cheese

1. Heat the oven to 400°F.

2. In a nonstick skillet over low heat, warm the oil and garlic until the garlic sizzles, about 1 minute. Add the spinach. Cook, tossing, until the spinach is wilted, about 2 minutes.

3. Set the tortilla on a baking sheet and sprinkle with Parmesan. Top with the spinach, then the chicken, bacon, and mozzarella. Bake for 7 to 10 minutes, or until the cheese is bubbly. Cut into wedges and serve.

Serves 1

PER SERVING: 405 calories, 35 g protein, 25 g carbs, 15 g fiber, 1 g sugar, 19 g fat, 7 g saturated fat, 692 mg sodium

Chicken Salad Sandwich

PREP TIME: 7 MINUTES • COOK TIME: 3 MINUTES

This recipe is a great use for leftover rotisserie chicken and replaces high-calorie mayo with yogurt and sour cream. Make it even leaner by serving it on greens and omitting the raisins.

2 teaspoons low-fat sour cream

2 teaspoons low-fat plain yogurt

1 teaspoon spicy brown mustard

3 ounces cooked chicken breast meat (from a rotisserie chicken), cubed

2 tablespoons finely chopped celery

2 tablespoons grated carrot

1 tablespoon pine nuts

1 tablespoon golden raisins

1 tablespoon finely chopped onion

Pinch of ground black pepper

2 slices of whole grain bread

1 leaf romaine lettuce

½ plum tomato, sliced

1. In a medium bowl, stir together the sour cream, yogurt, and mustard. Toss in the chicken, celery, carrot, pine nuts, raisins, onion, and pepper until coated.

2. Spread the chicken salad on 1 slice of bread. Add the lettuce leaf and tomato slices and top with another bread slice.

Serves 1

PER SERVING: 402 calories, 35 g protein, 38 g carbs, 7 g fiber, 14 g sugar, 12 g fat, 2 g saturated fat, 585 mg sodium

Mason Jar Citrus Chicken Salad

PREP TIME: 10 MINUTES • COOK TIME: 7 MINUTES

This fresh and fruity recipe is a refreshing, colorful spin on chicken salad. Grilling an extra chicken breast at dinner makes putting together this salad for lunch the next day super simple. You could also use rotisserie chicken.

2 tablespoons orange juice

2 tablespoons 2% plain Greek yogurt

1 teaspoon honey

1 clove garlic, minced

⅛ teaspoon dried thyme

1 cooked beet, peeled and shredded (canned or packaged in produce section)

2 tablespoons crumbled feta cheese

1 grilled boneless, skinless chicken breast half (4 ounces)

¼ cup fresh orange sections

2 tablespoons unsalted shelled pistachios, chopped

2 cups arugula

1. To a 1-quart mason jar, add the orange juice, yogurt, honey, garlic, and thyme. Screw on the lid and shake vigorously.

2. In the mason jar, layer the salad ingredients in the following order: beet, feta, chicken, oranges, pistachios, and arugula. Replace the lid and refrigerate until ready to take.

3. To eat, shake the jar into a bowl or onto a plate; that should be enough to coat the salad with the dressing. If not, gently toss with a fork.

Serves 1

PER SERVING: 398 calories, 36 g protein, 32 g carbs, 6 g fiber, 23 g sugar, 15 g fat, 5 g sat, 459 mg sodium

Steak Lettuce Wraps

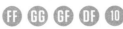

PREP TIME: 4 MINUTES • COOK TIME: 10 MINUTES

If you like steak and you like hummus, but have never tried them together, this tasty recipe will be a new favorite. Use a cast iron skillet if you're cooking indoors and don't have a grill pan.

1 teaspoon grated ginger

1 teaspoon olive oil

Pinch of salt

Pinch of ground black pepper

1 3-ounce piece skirt steak

2 tablespoons premade hummus

4 large romaine lettuce leaves

4 teaspoons pine nuts

1 scallion, sliced

½ cup fresh snow peas

1. Stir together the ginger, oil, salt, and pepper and brush onto the steak. Heat a grill or grill pan to medium and grill the steak until medium-rare, about 5 minutes. Slice the steak against the grain into strips.

2. Spread ½ tablespoon hummus on each of the lettuce leaves. Sprinkle with ½ teaspoon pine nuts and one-quarter of the scallion. Place one-quarter of the sliced steak and snow peas in each lettuce leaf, wrap, and serve.

Serves 1

PER SERVING: 350 calories, 25 g protein, 14 g carbs, 7 g fiber, 4 g sugar, 23 g fat, 4 g saturated fat, 481 mg sodium

Mason Jar Mediterranean Salad

PREP TIME: 7 MINUTES • COOK TIME: 10 MINUTES

Simple and delicious, this perfectly portable salad is a go-to for busy weeks. If you don't like olives, trade them for a few slices of avocado.

1 tablespoon olive oil

2 teaspoons lemon juice

¼ teaspoon dried oregano

Pinch of salt

Pinch of ground black pepper

½ medium cucumber, chopped

1 can (3 ounces) unsalted tuna in water, drained

¼ cup crumbled feta cheese

8 kalamata olives, pitted

1 medium tomato, chopped

2 cups baby spinach, rinsed

1. To a I-quart mason jar, add the olive oil, lemon juice, oregano, salt, and pepper. Screw on the lid and shake vigorously.

2. In the mason jar, layer the remaining ingredients in the following order: cucumber, tuna, feta, olives, tomato, and spinach. Replace the lid and refrigerate until ready to take.

3. To eat, shake the jar into a bowl or onto a plate; that should be enough to coat the salad with the dressing. If not, gently toss with a fork.

Serves 1

PER SERVING: 403 calories, 28 g protein, I4 g carbs, 4 g fiber, 6 g sugar, 27 g fat, 6 g saturated fat, 942 mg sodium

Healthy Egg Salad

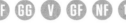

PREP TIME: 5 MINUTES • COOK TIME: 5 MINUTES

This recipe brings new flavor to classic egg salad, and the pumpkin seeds add a delightful crunch. Save the extra serving for lunch the next day, or enjoy lunch with a friend.

¼ cup 2% plain Greek yogurt

1 teaspoon Dijon mustard

2 sliced scallions

2 tablespoons golden raisins

2 tablespoons chia seeds

½ teaspoon curry powder (optional)

Salt and ground black pepper to taste

4 hard-cooked eggs, chopped

4 Bibb or butter lettuce leaves

½ avocado, sliced

2 tablespoons cilantro leaves

2 teaspoons pumpkin seeds

1. In a medium bowl, mix the yogurt, mustard, scallions, raisins, chia seeds, curry powder (if using), and salt and pepper to taste. Stir in the eggs.

2. In a I-quart mason jar, layer the lettuce with the egg mixture. Top with the avocado, cilantro, and pumpkin seeds. Cover with the lid and refrigerate until ready to eat.

3. To eat, shake the jar into a bowl or onto a plate.

Serves 2

PER SERVING: 372 calories, 20 g protein, 22 g carbs, 9 g fiber, IO g sugar, 24 g fat, 5 g saturated fat, 284 mg sodium

Sweet Potato Nachos

  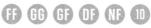

PREP TIME: 10 MINUTES • COOK TIME: 10 MINUTES

Nachos are notoriously high in calories and full of highly processed ingredients. This recipe replaces tortilla chips with crispy sweet potatoes to keep things clean. If you enjoy dairy, top with a sprinkle of feta or cotija cheese.

1 medium sweet potato, peeled and very thinly sliced

1 teaspoon olive oil

3 ounces ground beef or bison

1 teaspoon chili powder

1 teaspoon garlic powder

¼ teaspoon smoked paprika

¼ cup drained and rinsed canned black beans

1 plum tomato, chopped

¼ avocado, chopped

2 tablespoons cotija or feta cheese (optional)

1 scallion, chopped

1. Heat the oven to 425°F. Coat a foil-lined baking sheet with olive oil cooking spray. Lay the sweet potato slices in a single layer and coat with more cooking spray. Roast until crisp, about 10 minutes.

2. Meanwhile, in a medium skillet over medium heat, heat the oil. Add the beef or bison, chili powder, garlic powder, and paprika and cook, breaking the beef up with a wooden spoon, until browned, 5 minutes. Stir in the black beans to heat through.

3. Transfer the sweet potato chips to a plate and top with the beef and bean mixture, tomato, avocado, cheese (if using), and scallion.

Serves 1

PER SERVING: 425 calories, 24 g protein, 47 g carbs, 11 g fiber, 10 g sugar, 17 g fat, 4 g saturated fat, 330 mg sodium

Dijon Salmon Buckwheat Bowl

PREP TIME: 5 MINUTES • COOK TIME: 15 MINUTES

This recipe combines two superfoods—salmon and buckwheat—in one very simple dish. Buckwheat is a gluten-free seed that is cooked similarly to rice or quinoa and is a great, nutrient-rich substitute for any grain.

¼ cup buckwheat groats

½ cup water

6 ounces canned salmon packed in water, drained

2 tablespoons finely chopped flat-leaf parsley

1 tablespoon finely chopped shallot

1 tablespoon lemon juice

1 teaspoon Dijon mustard

Ground black pepper, to taste

½ cup steamed green beans, cut into 1-inch lengths

1. In a small saucepan, bring the buckwheat groats and water to a boil. Reduce the heat, cover, and cook until tender, about 10 minutes.

2. Meanwhile, toss together the salmon, parsley, shallot, lemon juice, mustard, and pepper.

3. Fluff the buckwheat with a fork and top with the salmon mixture and green beans.

Serves 1

PER SERVING: 375 calories, 41 g protein, 40 g carbs, 7 g fiber, 2 g sugar, 7 g fat, 1.5 g saturated fat, 670 mg sodium

Portobello Turkey Burger
with Bruschetta

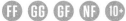

PREP TIME: 10 MINUTES • COOK TIME: 10 MINUTES

This recipe trades a whole wheat bun for portobello mushrooms. Use a cast iron skillet if you don't have access to a grill or grill pan.

4 ounces ground turkey

¼ teaspoon garlic powder

⅛ teaspoon kosher salt, plus more to taste

⅛ teaspoon ground black pepper, plus more to taste

2 large portobello mushrooms, wiped clean and stems removed

1 plum tomato, coarsely chopped

1 tablespoon chopped red onion

1 thinly sliced basil leaf

1 tablespoon balsamic vinegar

1 slice (½-ounce) fresh mozzarella cheese

1. In a small bowl, combine the turkey, garlic powder, salt, and pepper. Form into a patty.

2. Heat a grill or grill pan to medium high and lightly oil the grates. Cook the turkey burger and portobello caps, flipping once, until the burger is cooked through and the mushrooms are tender, about 8 minutes.

3. Meanwhile, in a small bowl, combine the tomato, onion, basil, and vinegar. Season to taste with salt and pepper.

4. Using the mushroom caps as buns, place the burger inside, top with the cheese and bruschetta mixture, and enjoy.

Serves 1

PER SERVING: 267 calories, 30 g protein, 13 g carbs, 3 g fiber, 9 g sugar, 12 g fat, 3.5 g saturated fat, 341 mg sodium

Chickpea-Lentil Tabbouleh

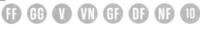

PREP TIME: 7 MINUTES • COOK TIME: 3 MINUTES

This recipe is ready to eat so quickly you won't believe how good it tastes. Allow it to chill in the fridge for a few hours to deepen the flavors.

- ¾ cup no-salt-added drained and rinsed canned chickpeas
- ½ cup no-salt-added drained and rinsed canned lentils
- ½ cup halved cherry tomatoes
- ¼ cup chopped flat-leaf parsley
- 2 tablespoons chopped mint
- 2 tablespoons chopped basil
- 2 tablespoons fresh lemon juice, plus more to taste
- 1 teaspoon extra-virgin olive oil

  Kosher salt and ground black pepper, to taste

1. In a medium bowl, combine the chickpeas, lentils, and tomatoes.

2. Add the parsley, mint, basil, lemon juice, olive oil, and salt and pepper to taste and stir to combine. Serve cold or at room temperature.

Serves 1

PER SERVING: 366 calories, 20 g protein, 58 g carbs, 18 g fiber, 6 g sugar, 7 g fat, 1 g saturated fat, 449 mg sodium

Rainbow Chard Chicken Wrap

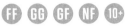

PREP TIME: 10 MINUTES • COOK TIME: 12 MINUTES

Swiss chard is mild in flavor, and the wide leaves make it an amazing alternative to tortillas and taco shells. Eat this healthy twist on a burrito with your hands or use a knife and fork to keep the delicious filling from spilling out the ends.

1 teaspoon olive oil

½ medium sweet potato, peeled and chopped

½ red bell pepper, chopped

½ medium onion, chopped

2 leaves rainbow chard, tough stems removed and chopped

Kosher salt and ground black pepper, to taste

4 ounces cooked chicken breast, sliced (about 1 cup)

2 tablespoons 2% plain Greek yogurt

1. In a medium skillet, heat the oil over medium heat. Add the sweet potato, bell pepper, onion, diced chard stems, and salt and pepper to taste. Cover the pan and cook, stirring occasionally, until the sweet potato is tender, about 8 minutes.

2. Spread the chard leaves on a work surface and divide the chicken between them. Top with the sweet potato mixture and a dollop of yogurt. Roll up the chard, tucking in the sides as you would a burrito. Secure with a toothpick, if necessary.

Serves 1

PER SERVING: 356 calories, 42 g protein, 25 g carbs, 6 g fiber, 11 g sugar, 10 g fat, 2 g saturated fat, 614 mg sodium

Chorizo and Calabaza Spanish Tortilla

PREP TIME: 5 MINUTES • COOK TIME: 10 MINUTES

Precooked Spanish sausage, chorizo, is sold at most supermarkets in the butcher's case. If they don't have the precooked stuff, don't worry. You can use the same amount of the fresh Mexican chorizo, but instead of dicing it, use it like ground beef and crumble and brown it in this recipe.

1½ ounces smoked
   chorizo, diced

¼ cup chopped onion

1 cup diced steamed
   pumpkin or
   butternut squash

2 large eggs

2 tablespoons whole milk

Ground black pepper

1. Spray a small skillet with nonaerosol cooking spray. Over medium heat, cook the chorizo and onion until the onion becomes translucent, about 2 minutes. Stir in the pumpkin or squash and distribute across the skillet.

2. In a small bowl, whisk together the eggs and milk until frothy. Pour over the chorizo and vegetables in the skillet and cover the skillet. Cook until the egg tortilla is set and puffy, about 5 minutes. Flip and cook until the eggs are lightly brown on the bottom, about 2 minutes more. Transfer to a plate and season to taste with the pepper.

Serves 1

PER SERVING: 402 calories, 25 g protein, 14 g carbs, 1 g fiber, 7 g sugar, 27 g total fat, 10 g saturated fat, 683 mg sodium

Miso Salmon with Green Tea Brown Rice

PREP TIME: 3 MINUTES • COOK TIME: 7 MINUTES

This recipe calls for brown rice, but you can swap in quinoa to keep it grain-free. Precooked brown rice or quinoa, either frozen or in the rice section, is a time-crunched cook's best friend. Some cook as fast as 90 seconds in the microwave.

1 skin-on salmon fillet (6 ounces), about ³⁄₄ inch thick

1 tablespoon organic white miso

2 teaspoons water

¹⁄₂ cup cooked brown rice

¹⁄₂ cup hot green tea (prepared according to package instructions)

2 tablespoons thinly sliced scallion

¹⁄₂ teaspoon toasted sesame seeds

1. Position a rack 4 inches from the broiler and heat the broiler on high. Line a baking sheet with foil.

2. Put the salmon skin-side down on the baking sheet. Broil for 2 minutes. Meanwhile, in a small bowl, stir the miso with the water to loosen. Spread the miso mixture over the top of the salmon and broil until the salmon is just barely opaque in the center (use a paring knife to check), 2 to 3 minutes more.

3. Place the brown rice in a mound in the center of a wide, shallow bowl. Pour the green tea around the rice. Using a spatula, lift the salmon from the baking sheet, leaving the skin behind, and place on top of the rice. Sprinkle with the scallion and sesame seeds.

Serves 1

PER SERVING: 397 calories, 38 g protein, 29 g carbs, 3 g fiber, l g sugar, 13 g total fat, 2 g saturated fat, 719 mg sodium

Yellow Lentil Salad

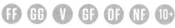

PREP TIME: 5 MINUTES • COOK TIME: 17 MINUTES

In addition to being rich in protein and other nutrients, lentils are inexpensive, making this a great recipe to quadruple when you want to feed a group. Adding a few handfuls of mixed greens will also help you bolster the recipe.

½ cup yellow lentils

2 cups water

1 tablespoon white wine vinegar

1½ teaspoons avocado oil

½ teaspoon lemon zest

½ teaspoon Dijon mustard

½ cup halved yellow cherry tomatoes

½ cup peeled and sliced cucumber

2 tablespoons chopped parsley

1 tablespoon shaved Parmesan cheese (optional)

1. Bring the lentils and water to a boil. Cook until the lentils are tender but not mushy, about 15 minutes.

2. Meanwhile, whisk together the vinegar, oil, zest, and mustard.

3. Toss the lentils with the tomatoes, cucumber, parsley, and the dressing. Top with the cheese, if using.

Serves 1

PER SERVING: 429 calories, 27 g protein, 61 g carbs, 16 g fiber, 5 g sugar, 9 g total fat, 1 g saturated fat, 98 mg sodium

Cuban-Style Pork Tenderloin with Black Bean Salad

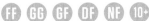

PREP TIME: 10 MINUTES • COOK TIME: 15 MINUTES

Bright flavor and hearty protein come together to create a meal that will keep you going all afternoon. Consider making an extra serving and eating it for lunch or dinner the next day.

1 tablespoon extra-virgin olive oil

½ small shallot, finely chopped

1 teaspoon distilled white vinegar

1 large clove garlic, minced

½ teaspoon chili powder

¼ teaspoon ground cumin

¼ teaspoon dried oregano

Kosher salt and ground black pepper, to taste

4 ounces pork tenderloin

½ cup drained and rinsed canned black beans

2 tablespoons chopped cilantro

2 tablespoons chopped red bell pepper

1 tablespoon fresh lime juice

1. In a small bowl, whisk together the oil, shallot, vinegar, garlic, chili powder, cumin, oregano, and salt and pepper to taste. Butterfly the tenderloin by cutting a lengthwise slit to within ½ inch of the other side of the tenderloin and open flat.

2. Spread the oil mixture all over the pork. Spray a medium skillet with nonaerosol cooking spray and cook the tenderloin until golden brown outside and slightly pink in the thickest parts (cut open to check), flipping once, about 5 minutes per side.

3. Meanwhile, combine the beans with the cilantro, red pepper, and lime juice. Season to taste with salt and pepper. Serve the pork over the black bean salad.

Serves 1

PER SERVING: 396 calories, 33 g protein, 33 g carbs, 8 g fiber, 3 g sugar, 17 g fat, 2.5 g saturated fat, 645 mg sodium

Shrimp and Broccoli Stir-Fry

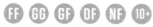

PREP TIME: 10 MINUTES • **COOK TIME:** 10 MINUTES

Chinese food is notoriously high in calories and full of additives. Clean it up and still get your fix with this simply delicious recipe.

2 teaspoons grapeseed oil

1 cup sliced red or orange bell pepper

½ cup sliced white onion

1 clove garlic, minced

3 cups small broccoli florets

2 tablespoons water

6 ounces peeled and deveined shrimp

1 tablespoon coconut aminos or low-sodium soy sauce

1 teaspoon toasted sesame oil

Ground black pepper

1. Heat a wok or skillet over medium heat. Swirl in the grapeseed oil. Toss in the bell pepper, onion, and garlic and cook until tender, about 3 minutes.

2. Stir in the broccoli and water. Cook, stirring, until the broccoli is bright green, about 3 minutes more.

3. Push all the vegetables around the edges of the pan and add the shrimp in the center. Cook until bright pink all over, about 3 minutes.

4. Stir everything together. Pour the coconut aminos or soy sauce, sesame oil, and a generous amount of black pepper over all. Toss to coat and serve.

Serves 1

PER SERVING: 399 calories, 36 g protein, 34 g carbs, II g fiber, 12 g sugar, 15 g fat, 2 g saturated fat, 1,300 mg sodium

Beef Kebabs with Chimichurri

PREP TIME: 10 MINUTES • COOK TIME: 15 MINUTES

Impress your guests with this delicious recipe. The colorful chimichurri sauce adds fresh flavor to protein-packed kebabs.

For the kebabs:

8 multicolored cherry tomatoes

6 ounces sirloin steak, cut into 6 even cubes

½ small red onion cut into 4 wedges

1 thick asparagus spear, trimmed and cut into quarters

4 1- to 2-inch cauliflower florets

Kosher salt and ground black pepper

For the chimichurri:

1 tablespoon chopped parsley

1 tablespoon chopped cilantro

1 small clove garlic, mashed

1 tablespoon red wine vinegar

1 tablespoon water

2 teaspoons extra-virgin olive oil

Kosher salt, to taste

Crushed red pepper flakes, to taste

1. To prepare the kebabs: Prepare a grill or grill pan on high heat. Skewer the kebab ingredients in the following order: tomato, beef cube, onion wedge, tomato, asparagus (horizontal), cauliflower, beef cube, onion wedge, tomato, asparagus, cauliflower, beef cube, tomato. Spray with nonaerosol cooking spray and season with salt and pepper. Repeat with another skewer.

2. Grill the kebabs, turning a few times, until the vegetables are tender and the meat is done to your liking, about 6 minutes total for medium-rare.

3. To make the chimichurri: Put the parsley, cilantro, garlic, vinegar, water, oil, salt, and pepper flakes in a jar, cap it, and shake to combine.

4. Let the kebabs rest on a plate a few minutes before drizzling with the chimichurri and serving.

Serves 1

PER SERVING: 422 calories, 41 g protein, 14 g carbs, 4 g fiber, 7 g sugar, 22 g fat, 5 g saturated fat, 607 mg sodium

Coconut-Crusted Chicken Fingers with Pineapple Salsa

(FF) (GG) (GF) (DF) (NF) (10+)

PREP TIME: 7 MINUTES • COOK TIME: 11 MINUTES

This recipe puts a healthy twist on a kid-friendly classic. Double or triple this and you'll happily eat the leftovers for lunch the next day.

5 chicken tenders

Kosher salt and ground black pepper, to taste

1 large egg

1 tablespoon water

½ cup shredded unsweetened coconut

½ cup finely chopped fresh pineapple

1 tablespoon finely chopped red onion

1 teaspoon chopped cilantro

1 teaspoon fresh lime juice

1. Heat the oven to 425°F. Line a baking sheet with foil and spray with nonaerosol cooking spray.

2. Season the chicken with salt and pepper. Beat the egg and water in a wide, shallow bowl. Place the coconut in another wide, shallow bowl. Dip the chicken in the egg, then in the coconut, and transfer to the prepared baking sheet. Bake until cooked through and the coconut is toasted, about 10 minutes.

3. Meanwhile, mix the pineapple, onion, cilantro, and lime juice. Season generously with black pepper.

4. Transfer the chicken to a plate and serve with the salsa.

Serves 1

PER SERVING: 407 calories, 19 g protein, 28 g carbs, 4 g fiber, 10 g sugar, 24 g fat, 10 g saturated fat, 732 mg sodium

Seared Tuna Sushi Bowl

PREP TIME: 5 MINUTES • COOK TIME: 5 MINUTES

This recipe calls for brown rice, but you can swap in quinoa to keep it grain-free. Precooked brown rice or quinoa, either frozen or in the rice section, will greatly cut down on your time in the kitchen. Also, make life easier by getting julienned carrots, available in the produce section. You may want to add wasabi paste or pickled ginger, but they have sugar in them, so try using wasabi powder and mix it yourself with some water and fresh grated ginger. You can find nori (sheets of dried seaweed) in the Asian section of most supermarkets.

½ cup cooked brown rice, warmed

1 teaspoon rice vinegar

1 teaspoon black sesame seeds

1½ teaspoons grapeseed oil

5 ounces high-quality, center-cut tuna steak

½ cup sliced and seeded cucumber

⅓ cup grated or julienned carrot

3 tablespoons thinly sliced nori

Wasabi paste, for serving (optional)

Grated ginger, for serving (optional)

1. In a bowl, combine the rice, vinegar, and sesame seeds. Cover and keep warm.

2. In a small nonstick skillet over medium heat, heat the oil. Add the tuna and sear, I minute per side. Transfer to a cutting board and slice about ¼ inch thick.

3. Top the rice with the tuna, cucumber, carrot, and nori. Serve with homemade wasabi paste and grated fresh ginger, if desired.

Serves 1

PER SERVING: 4I5 calories, 37 g protein, 29 g carbs, 4 g fiber, 3 g sugar, I6 g total fat, 3 g saturated fat, 84 mg sodium

Grilled Mushroom Burgers

PREP TIME: 8 MINUTES • COOK TIME: 12 MINUTES

These plant-based "burgers" are an awesome way to end the day. If you have a little more time, consider marinating the mushroom caps in a little vinegar, oil, basil, oregano, garlic, salt, and pepper prior to grilling.

- 4 large portobello mushroom caps, stems removed
- 1 large white onion, sliced into four ½-inch-thick rounds
- 2 tablespoons balsamic vinegar
- 1 cup roasted red bell pepper strips
- 4 100% whole wheat buns, halved
- 6 tablespoons premade pesto
- 2 tablespoons hulled hemp seeds
- 4 slices provolone cheese
- 1 cup spinach, rinsed

1. Heat a grill or grill pan over medium heat. Grill the mushrooms and onion slices until tender, 8 minutes, turning halfway during cooking and brushing with the vinegar. Warm the pepper strips and buns on the grill.

2. In a small bowl, stir together the pesto and hemp seeds. Divide the pesto mixture between each bun bottom. Top with a mushroom, 1 slice of onion, 1 slice of cheese, and one-quarter of the pepper strips. Place ¼ cup spinach leaves on top of each burger and cap with the bun top.

Serves 4

PER SERVING: 412 calories, 20 g protein, 35 g carbs, 6 g fiber, 10 g sugar, 23 g fat, 8 g saturated fat, 817 mg sodium

Spinach-Quinoa Bowl with Kale Pesto

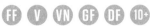

This plant-based recipe can be whipped up even faster by using jarred pesto and precooked quinoa. You also sub in more baby spinach for the kale if you prefer.

⅓ cup dry quinoa, rinsed

⅔ cup + 2 teaspoons water, divided

½ cup torn kale leaves

1 tablespoon raw almonds

1 tablespoon nutritional yeast flakes

1 tablespoon fresh lemon juice

1 teaspoon olive oil

1 clove garlic

¼ teaspoon kosher salt

¼ teaspoon ground black pepper

2 cups baby spinach, rinsed

¼ cup drained and rinsed canned white beans

1. Cook the quinoa in ⅔ cup water according to package instructions.

2. Meanwhile, in a food processor, pulse together the kale, almonds, nutritional yeast, lemon juice, 2 teaspoons water, olive oil, garlic, salt, and pepper until smooth.

3. When the quinoa is done cooking, raise the heat to medium and stir in the spinach, kale pesto, and white beans. Cook until the spinach is wilted and the beans and pesto are heated through. Transfer to a bowl and enjoy.

Serves 1

PER SERVING: 435 calories, 21 g protein, 62 g carbs, 13 g fiber, 4 g sugar, 14 g fat, 1.5 g saturated fat, 587 mg sodium

Arugula Salad with Zucchini Ribbons

PREP TIME: 5 MINUTES • COOK TIME: 5 MINUTES

This salad is heartier than it looks. The healthy fats from the olive oil and pumpkin seeds, plus the protein and fiber from the chickpeas, make for a light yet satisfying meal. Our test panelists were happily surprised by how delicious and filling it was.

3 tablespoons extra-virgin olive oil

Juice of ½ lemon

4 cups arugula

1 medium zucchini

1 can (15.5 ounces) chickpeas, drained and rinsed

1 cup artichoke hearts, drained and quartered

½ cup toasted pumpkin seeds

3 ounces (about ¾ cup) Parmesan cheese, shaved

1. In a large bowl, stir together the olive oil and lemon juice. Place the arugula in the bowl.

2. Over the arugula and using a vegetable peeler, shave the zucchini on one side over and over to make ribbons, turning every few strokes to distribute the peel evenly. Stop when you reach the seedy core and no more ribbons can be sliced.

3. Add the chickpeas and artichoke hearts and gently toss to coat with the dressing. Sprinkle with the pumpkin seeds and Parmesan shavings. Serve immediately.

Serves 2

PER SERVING: 408 calories, 20 g protein, 28 g carbs, 10 g fiber, 5 g sugar, 26 g fat, 7 g saturated fat, 366 mg sodium

Falafel with Lemony Yogurt Sauce

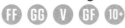

PREP TIME: 7 MINUTES • COOK TIME: 10 MINUTES

Homemade falafel is a treat that doesn't have to take a lot of time. This recipe offers the flavor of the traditional dish without wheat flour or deep-frying.

⅔ cup drained and rinsed canned chickpeas

1 clove garlic

½ medium onion, chopped

½ cup chopped parsley or cilantro

¼ teaspoon ground cumin

3 teaspoons fresh lemon juice, divided

Kosher salt and ground black pepper

¼ cup almond meal

¼ teaspoon baking powder

¼ cup 2% plain Greek yogurt

1 tablespoon chopped chives

1. In a blender, pulse the chickpeas and garlic until broken up. Add the onion, parsley or cilantro, cumin, I teaspoon of the lemon juice, and a pinch of salt and pepper and pulse until pasty but not pureed. Pulse in the almond meal and baking powder.

2. Lightly coat a large skillet with nonaerosol cooking spray and put over medium heat. Spoon golf ball–size portions of the mix into the skillet, gently press until flattened, and cook until golden and crispy on both sides, about 6 minutes total.

3. Meanwhile, mix together the yogurt, chives, and the remaining 2 teaspoons lemon juice. Serve alongside the falafel patties.

Serves 1

PER SERVING: 435 calories, 21 g protein, 54 g carbs, 12 g fiber, 6 g sugar, 18 g fat, 2 g saturated fat, 603 mg sodium

Black-Eyed Peas and Brown Rice Bowl

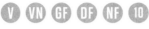

PREP TIME: 5 MINUTES • COOK TIME: 5 MINUTES

To make this rice bowl speedy, use frozen brown rice that only takes a few minutes to heat in the microwave. You can also use quinoa instead of brown rice if you prefer.

1 cup drained and rinsed canned black-eyed peas

½ cup cooked brown rice

¼ cup chopped roasted red peppers

2 teaspoons minced pickled jalapeños (or to taste)

1 teaspoon ground cumin

¼ avocado

2 tablespoons nutritional yeast flakes

2 teaspoons fresh lime juice

1 tablespoon cilantro leaves

1. In a medium microwaveable bowl, combine the black-eyed peas, rice, red peppers, jalapeños, and cumin. Cover and cook on high until heated through, about I minute.

2. In a separate bowl, smash together the avocado, nutritional yeast, and lime juice. Spoon on top of the rice mixture and sprinkle with the cilantro.

Serves 1

PER SERVING: 430 calories, 2I g protein, 73 g carbs, I7 g fiber, 2 g sugar, 7 g fat, I g saturated fat, 923 mg sodium

Almond-Encrusted Salmon with Greens

This salmon is so good that you'll happily eat any leftovers chilled on a salad or in a sandwich the next day.

¼ cup chopped almonds

¼ cup chopped flat-leaf parsley

1 tablespoon grated lemon zest

¼ teaspoon salt

Ground black pepper, to taste

1 large egg

2 skinless salmon fillets (4 ounces each)

2 tablespoons extra-virgin olive oil

4 cups mixed organic baby greens, spinach (rinsed), or watercress

Lemon wedges, for serving

1. Mix the almonds, parsley, lemon zest, salt, and black pepper in a wide, shallow bowl. Beat the egg in another wide, shallow bowl. Pat the salmon dry with a paper towel. Dip I salmon fillet into the egg, turning to coat. Transfer the fillet to the bowl with the almond mixture and press firmly so the almonds adhere. Set aside and repeat with the second fillet.

2. Warm the oil in a large skillet over medium heat. Add the salmon and cook, turning once, until it's opaque in the center (use a knife to check), 5 to 7 minutes.

3. Arrange 2 cups of greens per plate and place a cooked salmon fillet on top of the greens. Garnish with lemon wedges and serve immediately.

Serves 2

PER SERVING: 405 calories, 30 g protein, 7 g carbs, 4 g fiber, 2 g sugar, 29 g fat, 4 g saturated fat, 315 mg sodium

Poached Salmon
with Steamed Vegetables

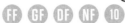

PREP TIME: 5 MINUTES • COOK TIME: 11 MINUTES

If you've never poached salmon, you're in for a treat. Simmering the delicate fish in a flavorful broth creates a lovely flavor and texture. And it doesn't take a lot of time! Use the leftovers to top salads or sandwiches.

6 cups water

1 celery stalk, quartered

1 lemon, sliced

4 skinless salmon fillets
(6 ounces each)

2 cups sugar snap peas

2 medium carrots,
sliced into coins

1 bunch asparagus,
ends trimmed

1. In a large pan with a lid, heat the water with the celery and lemon. Bring to a boil, reduce the heat, and add the salmon fillets (the water should just cover the fillets). Cover the pan and cook until the salmon is opaque, 8 to 10 minutes (depending on thickness).

2. Meanwhile, fill a large pot with 1 inch of water and put a steamer basket in the bottom. Bring to a boil and add the peas, carrots, and asparagus. Steam the vegetables until tender-crisp, about 5 minutes.

3. To serve, divide the vegetables among 4 plates. Carefully lift the salmon from the poaching liquid and place the salmon atop the vegetables (discard poaching liquid, celery, and lemon).

Serves 4

PER SERVING: 402 calories, 38 g protein, 9 g carbs, 3 g fiber, 5 g sugar, 23 g fat, 5 g saturated fat, 122 mg sodium

Speedy Fish Tacos

PREP TIME: 5 MINUTES • COOK TIME: 5 MINUTES

When you're short on time and craving Mexican, this recipe delivers. If you don't like spice, use plain diced tomatoes.

1 tablespoon olive oil

1 clove garlic, minced

½ teaspoon dried oregano

¼ teaspoon ground cumin

2 cans (6 ounces each) tuna packed in oil, drained and flaked

1 can (14 ounces) diced tomatoes with zesty jalapeños, well drained

¼ teaspoon hot pepper sauce

Juice of ½ lime

8 corn tortillas (6-inch diameter)

1 cup shredded low-fat Monterey Jack cheese

1. In a medium microwaveable dish, stir together the oil, garlic, oregano, and cumin. Microwave on high until heated through, about 60 seconds. Stir in the tuna, tomatoes, hot sauce, and lime juice. Microwave on high until heated through, about 2 minutes, stopping once to stir.

2. Warm the tortillas by wrapping them in a paper towel and microwaving them for 5 to 10 seconds. To serve, spoon some of the hot filling into each tortilla, top with 2 tablespoons of cheese, and fold up.

Serves 4

PER SERVING: 401 calories, 33 g protein, 29 g carbs, 4 g fiber, 5 g sugar, 18 g fat, 5 g saturated fat, 854 mg sodium

Chicken Stir-Fry

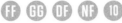

PREP TIME: 5 MINUTES • COOK TIME: 8 MINUTES

This easy-to-make dish is great for busy weekday nights. Sugar snap or snow peas are great alternatives to asparagus. If you avoid gluten, you can use liquid aminos in place of the soy sauce.

1 tablespoon reduced-sodium soy sauce

2 teaspoons honey

2 tablespoons sesame oil

1 bunch asparagus, ends trimmed and stalks cut into 1-inch pieces

1 cup broccoli florets

1 clove garlic, minced

10 ounces (about 2½ cups) sliced cooked chicken breast

4 cups cooked brown rice

1 tablespoon sesame seeds

1. In a small bowl, combine the soy sauce and honey. Set aside.

2. Heat the oil in a large skillet or wok over medium-high heat. Add the asparagus, broccoli, and garlic. Cook for 4 minutes, stirring frequently. Toss in the chicken and soy sauce mixture and heat thoroughly, 1 to 2 minutes.

3. Divide the rice among 4 bowls, top with the chicken mixture, and sprinkle with the sesame seeds.

Serves 4

PER SERVING: 418 calories, 34 g protein, 43 g carbs, 6 g fiber, 5 g sugar, 12 g fat, 2 g saturated fat, 213 mg sodium

Fish and Vinegar Chips

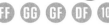

PREP TIME: 10 MINUTES • COOK TIME: 35 MINUTES

This recipe features two twists on the age-old classic: Crushed hazelnuts give a nice crunch to the oven-fried halibut in lieu of a deep-fried, flour-based batter, while root veggies (instead of the russet potato variety) pack in fiber and lots of flavor. To make this recipe as snappy as possible, get the veggies in the oven, then set to work on the fish; put the fish in the oven at about the same time that you toss the veggies so that everything's done at the same time.

1 pound mixed root vegetables (sweet potatoes, beets, carrots, turnips, and/or parsnips), peeled and cut into wedges

2 teaspoons olive oil

½ teaspoon kosher salt, divided

½ teaspoon ground black pepper, divided

1 tablespoon malt vinegar or apple cider vinegar plus more to serve (optional)

4 skinless halibut fillets (6 ounces each) or other white fish (cod, turbot, haddock)

¼ cup coconut flour

2 egg whites, beaten

¾ cup finely chopped hazelnuts or pecans

Lemon wedges (optional)

1. Heat the oven to 425°F. Line 2 large baking sheets with parchment paper.

2. Combine the vegetables, oil, half the salt, and half the black pepper in a large bowl, tossing well to coat. Arrange on one of the baking sheets in a single layer. Bake until browned and cooked through, turning once, about 30 minutes. Remove from the oven and toss with the vinegar.

3. Meanwhile, season the halibut with the remaining salt and pepper. Set the coconut flour, egg whites, and hazelnuts or pecans in their own separate shallow bowls. Working with I fillet at a time, dredge the halibut in the flour. Dip in the egg whites, shake off the excess, then roll in the nuts to coat. Place on the second baking sheet. Bake the halibut until the crumbs are golden brown and the fish flakes easily, turning once, about I2 minutes. (If the nuts start to brown too much, lay a piece of aluminum foil over the fish.)

4. Divide the fish and root vegetables among 4 plates. Serve with the lemon wedges and more malt vinegar, if desired.

Serves 4

PER SERVING: 4I2 calories, 39 g protein, 22 g carbs, 7 g fiber, 6 g sugar, I9 g fat, 3 g saturated fat, 423 mg sodium

Hearty Lasagna

PREP TIME: 5 MINUTES • COOK TIME: 45 TO 60 MINUTES

Get your Italian fix with this wheat-free version that uses zucchini in place of traditional noodles. Make sure to use a safety guard when slicing on the mandoline to protect your fingers.

3 cups whole-milk ricotta

½ cup chopped basil

3 links cooked chicken sausage, diced

2 large eggs

2 cloves garlic, minced

½ teaspoon red pepper flakes

2 medium zucchini

3 cups tomato basil pasta sauce, divided

3 tablespoons grated Parmesan cheese

1. Heat the oven to 350°F. Coat a 9" × 13" baking dish with nonaerosol cooking spray.

2. In a large bowl, mix together the ricotta, basil, sausage, eggs, garlic, and red pepper flakes.

3. Thinly slice the zucchini lengthwise using a mandoline or sharp knife. Spread ½ cup of the pasta sauce in the bottom of the prepared dish. Lay 4 zucchini "noodles" over the sauce, and cover with one-third of the ricotta mixture and 1 cup of the sauce. Repeat with another layer of zucchini, ricotta mixture, and sauce. Top with a final layer of zucchini, the remaining ricotta mixture, and ½ cup sauce. Sprinkle with Parmesan. Cover with foil and bake until the lasagna is heated through and bubbling, 30 to 45 minutes. Cool slightly before cutting and serving.

Serves 6

PER SERVING: 404 calories, 27 g protein, 20 g carbs, 3 g fiber, 9 g sugar, 25 g fat, 13 g saturated fat, 925 mg sodium

Pesto Chicken Bake

PREP TIME: 5 MINUTES • COOK TIME: 50 MINUTES

This recipe uses premade pesto to cut down on prep time. Using chicken thighs keeps this dish extra moist and juicy, but if you prefer white meat, use chicken breasts or tenders. If you have a busy week ahead, consider doubling the recipe and eating the leftovers throughout the week.

8 boneless, skinless chicken thighs

¼ teaspoon salt

¼ teaspoon ground black pepper

1 pound baby potatoes (red or Yukon Gold)

1 pint cherry tomatoes

⅓ cup premade pesto

2 tablespoons water

1 tablespoon olive oil

1. Heat the oven to 425°F. Season the chicken thighs with salt and pepper.

2. In a large roasting pan, combine the chicken thighs, potatoes, cherry tomatoes, pesto, water, and olive oil, gently tossing to coat all the ingredients with the pesto.

3. Bake until the potatoes are tender and the chicken is cooked through or an instant thermometer inserted in the thickest part reads 165°F, about 45 minutes. Serve 2 thighs with one-quarter of the veggies per person.

Serves 4

PER SERVING: 398 calories, 33 g protein, 24 g carbs, 4 g fiber, 3 g sugar, 19 g fat, 4 g saturated fat, 437 mg sodium

Chicken Tacos with Tangy Guacamole

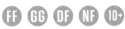

PREP TIME: 10 MINUTES • COOK TIME: 20 MINUTES

This recipe packs fresh flavors, lean protein, and healthy fat into one amazing dish. Top with diced tomatoes and sliced onion to dress it up, use lettuce wraps in place of tortillas to keep things grain-free, or create a taco salad.

1 small yellow onion, coarsely chopped

3 cloves garlic, halved

1 small serrano chile or jalapeño pepper, halved and seeded

$\frac{1}{2}$ cup loosely packed cilantro

Juice of 2 limes (about $\frac{1}{3}$ cup)

$\frac{1}{4}$ cup plus 1 tablespoon olive oil, divided

1 teaspoon salt, divided

$\frac{1}{4}$ teaspoon ground black pepper

4 boneless, skinless chicken breast halves (about $1\frac{1}{4}$ pounds)

2 ripe avocados

12 corn tortillas (6-inch diameter)

1. In a blender or food processor, blend the onion, garlic, chile pepper, cilantro, lime juice, $\frac{1}{4}$ cup olive oil, $\frac{1}{2}$ teaspoon salt, and black pepper until smooth. Put the chicken in a shallow dish and spread half of this mixture over all sides of the chicken and marinate for 10 minutes while you make the guacamole.

2. To make the guacamole: Peel and pit the avocados and put the flesh in a medium bowl. Add the remaining onion mixture and $\frac{1}{4}$ teaspoon salt. Coarsely mash with a fork and set aside, covered.

3. In a large skillet over medium heat, heat the remaining 1 tablespoon oil. Lift each chicken breast and let the excess marinade drip off (discard excess marinade). Add the chicken to the hot skillet and sprinkle with the remaining $\frac{1}{4}$ teaspoon salt. Brown on one side, about 5 minutes, then flip and finish cooking, 3 or 4 minutes longer. Remove to a cutting board and let rest 5 minutes before cutting against the grain into $\frac{1}{4}$-inch slices.

4. Wrap the tortillas in damp paper towels and microwave on high to warm them, 30 to 60 seconds. Serve the chicken with the tortillas and guacamole.

Serves 6

PER SERVING: 399 calories, 24 g protein, 28 g carbs, 7 g fiber, 1 g sugar, 22 g fat, 3 g saturated fat, 524 mg sodium

Spaghetti Squash Bolognese

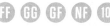

PREP TIME: 7 MINUTES • COOK TIME: 15 MINUTES

This recipe calls for turkey sausage, but you can also use lean ground beef or turkey. While this serves 1, it's easy to increase the amounts and make this for a group. No one will even miss the noodles! You can also use organic spaghetti sauce in place of the tomato puree if you're in a pinch. Just be sure it doesn't contain added sugar.

½ small spaghetti squash (about 3 pounds whole), halved lengthwise and seeded

1 teaspoon olive oil

3 ounces uncooked turkey sausage, casings removed

¼ cup chopped yellow onion

1 clove garlic, minced

1 teaspoon dried Italian seasoning

¼ teaspoon ground black pepper

¾ cup tomato puree

1 tablespoon 2% plain yogurt

Grated Parmesan cheese (optional)

1. Place the squash, cut side down, on a microwaveable plate. Cover with a microwaveable bowl and cook on high until the skin gives when lightly squeezed, about 10 minutes.

2. Meanwhile, heat the oil in a medium skillet over medium heat. Add the sausage, onion, garlic, Italian seasoning, and pepper. Cook, breaking up the sausage with a wooden spoon, until the sausage is no longer pink, about 5 minutes. Stir in the tomato puree and cook to meld the flavors, about 5 minutes more. Remove from the heat.

3. Remove the squash from the microwave and, using a fork, scrape out the strands. Toss the squash strands and yogurt into the sauce. Transfer to a plate and top with the cheese, if using.

Serves 1

PER SERVING: 379 calories, 23 g protein, 48 g carbs, 10 g fiber, 22 g sugar, 13 g fat, 3 g saturated fat, 639 mg sodium

Slow Cooker White Bean and Chicken Chili

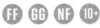

PREP TIME: 10 MINUTES • COOK TIME: 5 HOURS

This recipe stores in the fridge for up to a week, so you can enjoy it more than once. You can sub in ground chicken or turkey in place of the chicken breasts.

2 pounds boneless, skinless chicken breasts, cut into bite-size pieces

3 cans (15.5 ounces each) cannellini beans, drained and rinsed

1 quart reduced-sodium chicken broth

1 can (4.5 ounces) chopped green chile peppers with juice

2 onions, chopped

2 cloves garlic, minced

1 teaspoon ground cumin

¾ teaspoon dried oregano

½ teaspoon chili powder

½ teaspoon ground black pepper

½ teaspoon salt

⅛ teaspoon ground cloves

⅛ teaspoon cayenne pepper

¾ cup whole milk plain yogurt

Zest of 1 lime

2 tablespoons chopped cilantro leaves

1. Put the chicken, beans, broth, green chiles, onions, garlic, cumin, oregano, chili powder, black pepper, salt, cloves, and cayenne in a large slow cooker and stir well to combine. Cover and cook on low heat for 4 hours. Uncover and cook for I more hour, stirring occasionally.

2. Meanwhile, stir together the yogurt, lime zest, and cilantro. Serve the chili with a dollop of yogurt sauce.

Serves 6

PER SERVING: 357 calories, 42 g protein, 28 g carbs, 7 g fiber, 4 g sugar, 8 g fat, 2 g saturated fat, 790 mg sodium

Slow Cooker Stuffed Peppers

PREP TIME: 10 MINUTES • COOK TIME: 4 HOURS

This recipe uses quinoa in place of traditional rice and ground turkey instead of beef to result in a lean, protein-packed dinner you'll be happy to come home to at the end of a busy day. Consider freezing leftover peppers in individual, microwaveable containers; they take just a few minutes to defrost.

1 can (28 ounces) tomato puree

2 cups reduced-sodium chicken broth

½ teaspoon dried oregano

1 pound lean ground turkey

½ cup uncooked quinoa, rinsed

¼ cup chopped cilantro

3 scallions, chopped

1 small yellow onion, finely chopped

1 small jalapeño pepper, finely chopped

1 clove garlic, minced

¼ teaspoon salt

¼ teaspoon ground black pepper

4 large green bell peppers

2 tablespoons chopped parsley

2 tablespoons roasted salted pumpkin seeds

1. Combine the tomato puree, broth, and oregano in a slow cooker.

2. In a large bowl, combine the turkey, quinoa, cilantro, scallions, onion, jalapeño, garlic, salt, and black pepper. Cut the tops off the peppers and scoop out the seeds. Stuff each pepper with one-quarter of the turkey mixture. Replace the pepper tops and place in the slow cooker. Cover the slow cooker and cook on high heat for 4 hours or low for 8 hours.

3. To serve, carefully place I pepper into each of 4 bowls and spoon some sauce over and around them. Sprinkle each with 1½ teaspoons parsley and 1½ teaspoons pumpkin seeds.

Serves 4

PER SERVING: 409 calories, 34 g protein, 44 g carbs, 9 g fiber, 10 g sugar, 13 g fat, 3 g saturated fat, 322 mg sodium

Easy Slow Cooker Fajita Chicken

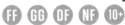

PREP TIME: 10 MINUTES • COOK TIME: 5 HOURS, 40 MINUTES

This is a fuss-free meal that your entire family will love. Using a few fresh spices instead of a packet of fajita seasoning eliminates artificial colorings and additives, making this a clean meal you can feel good about. To make this grain-free, use lettuce leaves in place of tortillas.

1 can (14.5 ounces) diced tomatoes

½ cup water

1 tablespoon chili powder

1 teaspoon ground cumin

1 teaspoon garlic powder

1 teaspoon salt

1 teaspoon ground black pepper

12 boneless, skinless chicken thighs

1 bag (12 ounces) frozen multicolored bell pepper strips

1 medium yellow onion, sliced

18 corn tortillas (6-inch diameter)

1 avocado, peeled and diced

1. In a slow cooker, stir together the tomatoes, water, chili powder, cumin, garlic powder, salt, and pepper. Add the chicken, pepper strips, and onion and stir to coat with the tomato mixture.

2. Cover and cook on low for 5 hours. Use 2 forks to shred the chicken, then cover and cook for 30 minutes more. Serve the chicken mixture with the corn tortillas, topping each with the avocado.

Serves 6

PER SERVING: 420 calories, 33 g protein, 45 g carbs, 9 g fiber, 4 g sugar, 13 g fat, 2 g saturated fat, 702 mg sodium

Slow Cooker Pork, Kale, and White Bean Soup

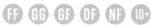

PREP TIME: 10 MINUTES • COOK TIME: 4 HOURS, 5 MINUTES

When you walk in the door after a busy day and smell this soup simmering, you'll be so glad you took a few minutes to throw it together earlier in the day. If desired, you can replace the ground pork with ground chicken.

1 tablespoon olive oil

1 pound lean ground pork

3 cloves garlic, minced

½ teaspoon dried thyme

½ teaspoon fennel seeds

¼ teaspoon dried sage

1 white onion, diced

3 carrots, diced

2 ribs celery, diced

4 cups reduced-sodium chicken broth

2 cups water

1 bay leaf

½ teaspoon kosher salt

½ teaspoon ground black pepper

2 cans (15 ounces each) white beans (such as cannellini or great Northern), drained and rinsed

3 cups chopped kale or baby kale

1. In a large skillet over medium-high heat, heat the olive oil. Add the pork and cook, breaking it up with a wooden spoon, until lightly browned, about 4 minutes. Add the garlic, thyme, fennel, and sage and cook until fragrant, 1 minute more.

2. Transfer the mixture to a 6-quart slow cooker along with the onion, carrots, celery, broth, water, bay leaf, salt, and pepper. Cover and cook until the vegetables are tender, on high for about 3½ hours or on low for about 7½ hours.

3. Stir in the beans and kale. Cover and cook until the kale is wilted and the beans are warmed through, about 30 minutes more. Remove the bay leaf before serving.

Serves 4

PER SERVING: 349 calories, 36 g protein, 35 g carbs, 10 g fiber, 6 g sugar, 9 g fat, 2 g saturated fat, 747 mg sodium

Lamb, Kale, and Sweet Potato Skillet

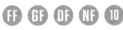

PREP TIME: 7 MINUTES • COOK TIME: 5 TO 6 MINUTES

To grate the sweet potato, use the large holes on a box grater (save time by making peeling optional) or use the grating blade on a food processor. Butternut squash would also work in this recipe. Swap out the kale for spinach for extra iron or beet greens for twice the fiber.

1 teaspoon olive oil

¼ pound ground lamb or beef

2 cups torn kale or baby kale

1 small sweet potato, grated (about ¾ cup)

2 tablespoons finely chopped onion

2 cloves garlic, minced

¼ teaspoon kosher salt

¼ teaspoon ground cumin

⅛ teaspoon crushed red pepper flakes

Chopped parsley, for garnish

1. In a nonstick skillet over medium heat, warm the oil. Add the lamb or beef and cook, breaking it up with a wooden spoon, until the lamb or beef is no longer pink, 3 to 4 minutes.

2. Add the kale, sweet potato, onion, garlic, salt, cumin, and pepper flakes. Cook until the kale and sweet potato are tender, about 2 minutes more. Serve sprinkled with the parsley.

Serves 1

PER SERVING: 397 calories, 27 g protein, 28 g carbs, 5 g fiber, 5 g sugar, 21 g fat, 7 g saturated fat, 618 mg sodium

Grilled Steak and Avocado Tacos

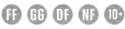

PREP TIME: 5 MINUTES • COOK TIME: 10 MINUTES

This recipe easily satisfies your craving for Mexican food. Replace the tortillas with lettuce leaves to make this grain-free.

Juice of 1 lime

2 cloves garlic, minced

1 tablespoon ground cumin

½ teaspoon red pepper flakes

½ teaspoon salt, plus more to taste

1 pound flank steak

1 ripe avocado, peeled and cubed

½ cup prepared salsa verde

1 scallion, sliced

2 tablespoons chopped cilantro

8 corn tortillas (6-inch diameter)

1. In a small bowl, stir together the lime juice, garlic, cumin, red pepper flakes, and salt. Rub all over the flank steak.

2. Heat a grill or grill pan to medium-high. Grill the steak to desired doneness, about 4 minutes per side for medium-rare. Transfer the steak to a cutting board and let stand for 5 minutes before cutting, against the grain, into thin strips.

3. Meanwhile, in a small bowl, combine the avocado, salsa verde, scallion, and cilantro. Season to taste with salt and set aside.

4. Warm the tortillas by wrapping them in a paper towel and microwaving them for 5 to 10 seconds. Serve with the steak and the avocado salsa.

Serves 4

PER SERVING: 394 calories, 28 g protein, 30 g carbs, 7 g fiber, 2 g sugar, 18 g fat, 5 g saturated fat, 548 mg sodium

Broiled Steak and Smashed Potatoes

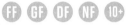

PREP TIME: 5 MINUTES • COOK TIME: 20 MINUTES

Surprise! You can eat steak and potatoes and still lose stubborn pounds. This recipe can easily be doubled if you're cooking for more than one. To change things up, use broccoli or Brussels sprouts in place of the green beans or asparagus.

4 ounces baby potatoes

¼ pound flank steak

4 ounces green beans or asparagus, ends trimmed

½ cup cherry tomatoes

2 teaspoons olive oil

¼ teaspoon salt

¼ teaspoon ground black pepper

1. Place the potatoes in a microwaveable bowl and cover with a microwaveable plate. Microwave on high until tender, about 8 minutes.

2. Heat the broiler to high. Line a baking sheet with aluminum foil and coat with nonaerosol cooking spray.

3. Arrange the steak, baby potatoes, green beans or asparagus, and cherry tomatoes on the prepared sheet. Brush or rub some of the oil on the steak, then toss the vegetables with the remaining oil. Sprinkle with the salt and pepper.

4. With the bottom of a glass, gently press the potatoes to flatten. Broil, flipping everything once, until the steak is cooked to your desired doneness, about 6 minutes for medium-rare. Remove from the oven and let rest for 5 minutes before slicing the steak against the grain.

Serves 1

PER SERVING: 373 calories, 28 g protein, 31 g carbs, 7 g fiber, 8 g sugar, 16 g fat, 4 g saturated fat, 660 mg sodium

Tex-Mex Sweet Potato

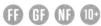

PREP TIME: 5 MINUTES • COOK TIME: 10 MINUTES

This recipe skips the high-sodium packets of taco seasoning and uses three simple ingredients already living in your spice cabinet. Save time by keeping a batch already mixed in a spice jar. Just double or quadruple the chili powder, cumin, and black pepper, and store in an airtight container for up to 6 months.

1 medium sweet potato

1 teaspoon olive oil

3 ounces ground beef (90% lean) or ground turkey

¼ medium onion, finely chopped

¼ cup fat-free refried beans

¼ cup fresh or frozen corn kernels

1 tablespoon chili powder

1 teaspoon ground cumin

½ teaspoon ground black pepper

1 tablespoon 2% plain Greek yogurt

¼ scallion (green or white part), sliced

1. Prick the potato all over with a fork to allow steam to escape. Place on a microwaveable plate and microwave on high until tender, 5 to 10 minutes.

2. Meanwhile, heat the oil in a medium skillet over medium heat. Add the beef or turkey and onion and cook, breaking up with a wooden spoon, until the beef is no longer pink and the onion has softened, 4 to 5 minutes. Add the refried beans, corn, chili powder, cumin, and black pepper, stirring to combine. Cook to meld the flavors, 1 minute more. Remove from the heat.

3. When cool enough to handle, cut the sweet potato in half lengthwise. Scoop the flesh out of the peel, leaving a thin layer of potato inside. Stir the flesh into the meat mixture.

4. Spoon the meat mixture into the potato-skin shells, mounding if necessary. Dollop with the yogurt and sprinkle with the scallion.

Serves 1

PER SERVING: 440 calories, 25 g protein, 58 g carbs, 9 g fiber, 10 g sugar, 13 g fat, 4 g saturated fat, 388 mg sodium

Cranberry Ginger Granola Bites

PREP TIME: 2 MINUTES • COOK TIME: 8 MINUTES, PLUS STANDING TIME

These homemade power bars are a delicious way to satisfy a craving for sweets. Store them in an airtight container or wrap individual servings and freeze them so they're fresh when you need a quick snack. Twenty seconds in the microwave is all it takes to quickly thaw them. If you avoid dairy, sub in plant-based protein powder.

- ¾ cup almond butter
- ½ cup pitted dates
- 2 scoops unsweetened vanilla whey protein powder
- ¼ teaspoon ground ginger
- 2 cups rolled oats
- ½ cup chopped almonds
- ¾ cup unsweetened dried cranberries

  Flaky sea salt, to garnish (optional)

1. Line an 8" x 8" baking pan with parchment paper.

2. In a food processor, pulse the almond butter, dates, protein powder, and ginger until smooth. Transfer to a medium bowl. Add the oats, almonds, and cranberries and knead until well combined. Press into the prepared pan (dampen hands if the mixture sticks). Sprinkle with the salt, if using.

3. Let stand until firm, about 2 hours. Slice into 16 pieces.

Serves 16 (1 bite each)

PER SERVING: 172 calories, 8 g protein, 16 g carbs, 4 g fiber, 5 g sugar, 10 g fat, 1 g saturated fat, 33 mg sodium

Beefed-Up Trail Mix

    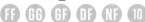

PREP TIME: 3 MINUTES • COOK TIME: 2 MINUTES

Beef jerky in trail mix? Once you try it, you'll never have it any other way. Opt for grass-fed beef jerky or organic turkey jerky that is low in added sugar.

- 2 cups air-popped popcorn
- 1 ounce organic, grass-fed beef jerky, chopped
- ¼ cup salted pepitas
- 2 tablespoons unsweetened dried cranberries, chopped

In a bowl, combine the popcorn, beef jerky, pepitas, and cranberries. Mix well.

Serves 2

PER SERVING: 182 calories, 10 g protein, 12 g carbs, 3 g fiber, 2 g sugar, 11 g fat, 3 g saturated fat, 331 mg sodium

Green Hummus and Veggies

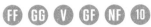

PREP TIME: 5 MINUTES • COOK TIME: 5 MINUTES

This recipe makes enough for a group or for a few days of snacking. If you're on the go, pack the hummus in the bottom of a mason jar, sprinkle with sunflower kernels, then sink the veggies upright into the hummus. Screw on the top and take it along!

1 can (15.5 ounces) chickpeas, drained and rinsed

½ cup chopped kale

¼ cup full-fat plain Greek yogurt

Juice of 1 lemon

1 tablespoon chia seeds

1 tablespoon tahini

Salt and ground black pepper, to taste

2 tablespoons sunflower kernels

8 asparagus spears, ends trimmed

1 cup broccoli florets

1 medium carrot, cut into sticks

Place the chickpeas, kale, yogurt, lemon juice, chia seeds, and tahini in a food processor and process until smooth. If necessary, add water by the tablespoon to thin. Season to taste with salt and pepper and transfer to a dish. Sprinkle with the sunflower kernels and serve with the vegetables.

Serves 4

PER SERVING: 154 calories, 9 g protein, 18 g carbs, 6 g fiber, 2 g sugar, 7 g fat, 1 g saturated fat, 257 mg sodium

Red Lentil Dip and Veggies

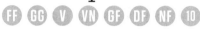

PREP TIME: 5 MINUTES • **COOK TIME:** 5 MINUTES

This fiber- and protein-packed dip is a clean alterative to the processed veggie dips you normally see at parties. Garam masala is a flavorful blend of Indian spices that adds a warm, sweet flavor. If you don't have it on hand, you can leave it out.

2 tablespoons parsley leaves

1 clove garlic

1 cup cooked red lentils

2 tablespoons fresh lemon juice

1 tablespoon coconut oil

½ teaspoon kosher salt

½ teaspoon garam masala (optional)

Your favorite cut vegetables, for dipping

1. In a food processor, pulse together the parsley and garlic until finely chopped.

2. Add the lentils, lemon juice, oil, salt, and garam masala (if using) and blend until smooth. Transfer to a bowl and enjoy with your favorite veggies.

Serves 2

PER SERVING, DIP ONLY: 179 calories, 9 g protein, 22 g carbs, 8 g fiber, 2 g sugar, 7 g fat, 6 g saturated fat, 483 mg sodium

Banana Peanut Butter "Ice Cream" Parfait

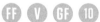

PREP TIME: 2 MINUTES • **COOK TIME:** 5 MINUTES

When you need an ice cream fix, this recipe will satisfy your craving naturally. You can sub the peanuts and nut butter with their almond equivalents. If you don't have blackberries, try strawberries or raspberries.

½ frozen medium banana

¼ cup fat-free plain Greek yogurt

1 teaspoon natural peanut butter

½ cup blackberries

Place the banana in a blender and blend until smooth, about 1 minute. In a small bowl, stir together the yogurt and peanut butter. In a parfait glass, alternate layers of banana with the yogurt mixture. Top with blackberries and serve.

Serves 1

PER SERVING: 148 calories, 9 g protein, 24 g carbs, 6 g fiber, 13 g sugar, 4 g fat, 1 g saturated fat, 25 mg sodium

Pear Wrapped in Cheddar and Prosciutto

  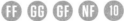

PREP TIME: 5 MINUTES • COOK TIME: 5 MINUTES

When you're entertaining, this recipe delivers a fast and easy appetizer that's sure to impress. Use a toothpick to keep each piece together or simply roll up this tasty treat, and opt for organic meats and cheeses whenever possible.

1 ounce thinly sliced prosciutto

½ ounce aged white Cheddar cheese, shredded

½ medium pear, cut lengthwise into 4 wedges

1. Cut the prosciutto into 4 strips and sprinkle the cheese on each.

2. Place a pear wedge on the edge of the prosciutto and roll up. Repeat with remaining pear and prosciutto.

Serves 1

PER SERVING: 169 calories, 12 g protein, 15 g carbs, 3 g fiber, 9 g sugar, 8 g fat, 4 g saturated fat, 848 mg sodium

Cocoa Ricotta Cup

   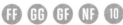

PREP TIME: 1 MINUTE • COOK TIME: 2 MINUTES

This recipe offers one of the fastest ways to satisfy your sweet tooth without reaching for highly processed junk. Opt for organic ricotta cheese or you might also whip this up with Greek yogurt.

½ cup fat-free ricotta cheese

1 tablespoon unsweetened natural cocoa powder

2 teaspoons maple syrup

½ teaspoon pure vanilla extract or finely grated orange zest

In a medium bowl, beat together the ricotta, cocoa powder, maple syrup, and vanilla extract with a wooden spoon until thoroughly combined. Transfer to a bowl and enjoy.

Serves 1

PER SERVING: 154 calories, 11 g protein, 22 g carbs, 2 g fiber, 13 g sugar, 1 g fat, 0.5 g saturated fat, 133 mg sodium

Raspberry Frozen Yogurt

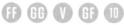

PREP TIME: 2 MINUTES • COOK TIME: 5 MINUTES

Blending frozen fruit with Greek yogurt creates a healthy ice cream–like treat in minutes. Feel free to swap your favorite berry for the raspberries!

¾ cup unsweetened frozen raspberries

½ cup 2% plain Greek yogurt

1 tablespoon chopped almonds

In a blender, pulse the raspberries until finely chopped. Add the yogurt and blend until smooth, about I minute. Transfer to a bowl, top with the almonds, and serve immediately.

Serves 1

PER SERVING: I50 calories, I2 g protein, I6 g carbs, 4 g fiber, 8 g sugar, 6 g fat, 2 g saturated fat, 38 mg sodium

Spiced "Baked" Apple with Yogurt

PREP TIME: 5 MINUTES • COOK TIME: 5 MINUTES

This recipe smells so good—the only thing better than the aroma is eating it! If you find yourself with extra time on your hands, this dish can also be done in an 8" × 8" baking dish, sprayed with nonaerosol cooking spray, then baked in a 375°F oven for about 30 minutes.

1 medium apple, halved and cored

½ teaspoon pumpkin pie spice

⅓ cup 2% plain Greek yogurt

1 teaspoon chia seeds

¼ teaspoon vanilla extract

⅛ teaspoon kosher salt

1. In a microwaveable dish, arrange the apple halves, skin sides down.

2. Sprinkle the apples with the pumpkin pie spice. Cover the dish with a microwaveable dome lid or damp paper towel. Microwave on high until the apple is tender, 3 to 4 minutes.

3. Meanwhile, stir together the yogurt, chia seeds, vanilla, and salt. Serve the cooked apple with the yogurt.

Serves 1

PER SERVING: I68 calories, 7 g protein, 30 g carbs, 6 g fiber, 22 g sugar, 3 g fat, I.5 g saturated fat, 268 mg sodium

Bananaberry "Pudding"

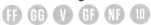

PREP TIME: 5 MINUTES • COOK TIME: 5 MINUTES

Use your favorite berries—blueberries, raspberries, or sliced strawberries—in this simple recipe. Opt for organic ricotta cheese when possible.

½ ripe banana

⅓ cup reduced-fat ricotta cheese

1 teaspoon ground cinnamon

¼ cup berries

In a bowl, mash the banana with a fork. Stir in the ricotta and cinnamon. Top with the berries and serve.

Serves 1

PER SERVING: 194 calories, 10 g protein, 25 g carbs, 4 g fiber, 11 g sugar, 7 g fat, 4 g saturated fat, 105 mg sodium

Wasabi Tuna Lettuce Wraps

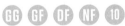

PREP TIME: 5 MINUTES • COOK TIME: 7 MINUTES

This recipe is big on flavor and low in carbs and added sugar. Store the extra serving in an airtight container and save it for tomorrow's afternoon snack.

1 can (about 5 ounces) water-packed tuna, drained

2 tablespoons chopped shallot

2 tablespoons rice vinegar

2 teaspoons reduced-sodium tamari or coconut aminos

1 teaspoon sesame oil

¼ teaspoon wasabi paste

4 Boston Bibb lettuce leaves, washed and dried

¼ cup thinly sliced scallion

½ teaspoon toasted sesame seeds

1. In a small bowl, combine the tuna, shallot, vinegar, tamari or aminos, sesame oil, and wasabi paste. Let sit for 5 minutes to meld the flavors.

2. Pile into the lettuce leaves and top with the scallion and sesame seeds.

Serves 2

PER SERVING: 141 calories, 15 g protein, 4 g carbs, 1 g fiber, 2 g sugar, 6 g fat, 1.5 g saturated fat, 435 mg sodium

Blueberry-Hazelnut Yogurt Bark

FF V GF 10+

PREP TIME: 3 MINUTES • COOK TIME: 3 HOURS 10 MINUTES

This frozen yogurt bark is sweet and refreshing. Consider making extra and storing it in the freezer in an airtight container. If you don't have or like hazelnuts, you can use a nut of your choice.

½ cup 2% plain
Greek yogurt

2 tablespoons wild
blueberries

1 tablespoon chopped
hazelnuts

1 teaspoon honey

1. Line a small baking dish with parchment paper.

2. In a small bowl, mix together the yogurt, blueberries, hazelnuts, and honey.

3. Spread the mixture in an even, ¼-inch-thick layer in the prepared dish and freeze until hard, about 3 hours.

4. Let sit at room temperature for a few minutes before breaking into bite-size pieces.

Serves 1

PER SERVING: 153 calories, 11 g protein, 14 g carbs, 1 g fiber, 12 g sugar, 7 g fat, 2 g saturated fat, 39 mg sodium

Chili Lime Crunchy Chickpeas

FF GG V VN GF DF NF 10

PREP TIME: 3 MINUTES • COOK TIME: 6 MINUTES

Make a double batch of these (using the whole can of chickpeas), because you're going to want them for a second snack! The chili powder lends warmth to the chickpeas, but if you think it may be too much for little palates, simply omit it.

1 teaspoon coconut oil

¾ cup drained and rinsed
canned chickpeas

1 teaspoon lime zest

½ teaspoon chili powder

¼ teaspoon kosher salt

1. In a medium skillet over medium-high heat, melt the oil. Add the chickpeas and cook until beginning to color, 3 to 4 minutes.

2. Stir in the lime zest, chili powder, and salt and cook until fragrant, 1 minute. Remove from the heat and let cool. The chickpeas will become crunchy as they cool.

Serves 1

PER SERVING: 198 calories, 9 g protein, 25 g carbs, 8 g fiber, 0 g sugar, 8 g fat, 4 g saturated fat, 981 mg sodium

Cacio e Pepe Popcorn

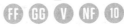

PREP TIME: 3 MINUTES • COOK TIME: 5 MINUTES

This healthful spin on the classic Roman pasta dish delivers a satisfyingly cheesy punch, thanks to the addition of nutritional yeast, which has zero saturated fat.

1 tablespoon coconut oil

½ cup popcorn kernels

2 tablespoons grated Parmesan cheese

2 tablespoons nutritional yeast flakes

1½ teaspoons ground black pepper

1 teaspoon kosher salt

1. In a pot over medium-high heat, melt the coconut oil. Add the popcorn kernels. Cover the pot and shake until the popping stops, 3 to 5 minutes.

2. Transfer the popcorn to a large bowl and toss in the Parmesan, nutritional yeast, pepper, and salt.

Serves 3

PER SERVING: 194 calories, 8 g protein, 25 g carbs, 6 g fiber, 0 g sugar, 7 g fat, 5 g saturated fat, 727 mg sodium

Brussels Sprouts Chips

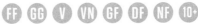

PREP TIME: 10 MINUTES • COOK TIME: 50 MINUTES

This recipe is kind of addicting, so consider doubling or tripling it so you can keep some on hand for a healthy snack. A food processor makes quick work of slicing the sprouts.

1 tablespoon reduced-sodium tamari or coconut aminos

1 teaspoon olive oil or coconut oil

¾ teaspoon maple syrup

¼ teaspoon garlic powder

10 ounces (about 2 cups) Brussels sprouts, trimmed and very thinly sliced

1. Heat the oven to 275°F and coat 2 baking sheets with non-aerosol cooking spray or line with parchment paper.

2. In a large bowl, whisk together the tamari, oil, maple syrup, and garlic powder. Add the sprouts and toss to coat. Let stand for 10 minutes for the flavors to absorb.

3. Scatter the slices in a single layer on the baking sheets. Bake, rotating the sheets halfway through, until the edges begin to brown and dry out, 35 to 40 minutes. (To test crispiness, let a chip cool on the counter for 30 seconds and taste.)

4. Let cool a bit before serving (they'll crisp up as they sit). Store the cooled chips in an airtight container at room temperature for up to 1 week.

Serves 1

PER SERVING: 178 calories, 11 g protein, 28 g carbs, 10 g fiber, 9 g sugar, 5 g fat, 1 g saturated fat, 683 mg sodium

Strawberry-Chia Kefir Pudding

(FF) (GG) (V) (GF) (NF) (10+)

PREP TIME: 5 MINUTES • COOK TIME: 1 HOUR, 5 MINUTES

The I-hour refrigeration gives the chia seeds time to expand and gel, giving this a pudding-like texture. Feel free to swap in a different-milk kefir if you are sensitive to cow's milk.

⅓ cup sliced strawberries

1 cup plain whole-milk kefir

1 teaspoon chia seeds

Mixed berries for serving (optional)

1. In a small bowl, mash the strawberries with a fork.

2. Add the kefir and chia seeds, stirring to combine. Cover and refrigerate for I hour or more before serving.

Serves 1

PER SERVING: I95 calories, II g protein, I8 g carbs, 2 g fiber, I5 g sugar, 9 g fat, 5 g saturated fat, I26 mg sodium

Kale Chips

(FF) (GG) (V) (VN) (GF) (DF) (NF) (10+)

PREP TIME: 5 MINUTES • COOK TIME: 17 MINUTES

If you love savory, crunchy snacks, you'll love this recipe. Be sure to buy nutritional yeast that comes in flake form, not the granules that are sometimes also called brewer's yeast. And make sure to keep an eye on the oven—kale chips have a tendency to go from not done to way-too-done very quickly.

3 cups coarsely chopped kale (tough ribs removed)

1 teaspoon grapeseed oil

1½ teaspoons nutritional yeast flakes

⅛ teaspoon salt

⅛ teaspoon ground black pepper

1. Heat the oven to 350°F. Lightly spray a baking sheet with nonaerosol cooking spray or line it with parchment paper.

2. In a large bowl, toss the kale with the grapeseed oil. Sprinkle with the nutritional yeast, salt, and pepper. Arrange the kale in a single layer on the baking sheet. Bake until crisp, about I5 minutes, tossing once. Serve immediately.

Serves 1

PER SERVING: I52 calories, II g protein, I9 g carbs, 5 g fiber, 0 g sugar, 7 g fat, 0.5 g saturated fat, 3I8 mg sodium

Savory Watermelon Salad

PREP TIME: 10 MINUTES • COOK TIME: 5 MINUTES

Who says salads can't be snacks? This one hits all the right sweet, savory, and crunchy notes.

½ cup 2% plain
  Greek yogurt

2 tablespoons fresh
  lemon juice

1 tablespoon chopped dill

1 tablespoon chopped mint

1 clove garlic, crushed
  in a press

¼ teaspoon kosher salt

¼ teaspoon ground
  black pepper

½ cup chopped watermelon

½ cup chopped cucumber

½ cup halved cherry
  tomatoes

2 tablespoons diced
  red onion

1 tablespoon roasted
  salted pistachios

1. In a small bowl, whisk together the yogurt, lemon juice, dill, mint, garlic, salt, and pepper.

2. Combine the watermelon, cucumber, tomatoes, and onion in a pint jar. Pour over the yogurt sauce, sprinkle with the pistachios, and seal with the lid. Shake it up and enjoy!

Serves 1

PER SERVING: 186 calories, 13 g protein, 23 g carbs, 3 g fiber, 14 g sugar, 6 g fat, 2 g saturated fat, 566 mg sodium

Acknowledgments

This book would never have been possible without an amazingly talented group of people. First, I want to thank the *Prevention* staff, including Editor-in-Chief Barbara O'Dair and Creative Director Courtney Murphy, for all that they've done to make Fit in 10 a success. I also want to thank Adam Campbell for believing in Fit in 10, and for launching me on this journey. I'm forever grateful for the opportunity to share Fit in 10 with the millions of busy women who are struggling to find a way to take care of themselves and their families. It's a blessing that I don't take lightly and a gift to do what I love.

I also must thank the core "Fit in 10 team." First, my editor, Erica Sanders-Foege, who helped me shape my initial ideas into the amazing book you now hold in your hands. Her experience elevated every aspect of this project, and I'm grateful for her guidance. This project also wouldn't have been possible without Art Director Carol Angstadt, who made every page beautiful, useful, and inviting and who has helped shape the visual look of the Fit in 10 brand since its inception. This project also wouldn't have been possible without Larysa DiDio, who has brought her sparkling energy and enthusiasm to Fit in 10 from the very beginning. Her talent and humor have helped to make the Fit in 10 workouts as enjoyable to do as they are effective. Editorial assistants Kasey Benjamin and Leah Polakoff also brought their excitement and commitment to this project, and I wouldn't have made it through this process nearly as easily without their valuable contributions. Thank you to Julissa Roberts and Jennifer Kushnier, who worked incredibly hard to develop the delicious 10-minute recipes.

Of course, there are so many other amazing people who have contributed to Fit in 10 along the way. To all of the photographers, designers, copy editors, and anyone else I didn't have room to mention here: Thank you from the bottom of my heart.

I also cannot say enough about the Fit in 10 test panelists who shared their stories: Each and every one of you is amazing, and I am so grateful I had the chance to get to know you! It's a true joy to watch you grow stronger, healthier, and leaner.

Last, to my friends and family who support and encourage me daily: Thank you! I love you and I am blessed to have you in my life.

Endnotes

LIFE IS COMPLICATED. FIT IN 10 IS SIMPLE.

1   US Department of Health and Human Services, Centers for Disease Control and Prevention, and National Center for Health Statistics, "Health Behaviors of Adults: United States, 2008–2010" (May 2013), http://www.cdc.gov/nchs/data/series/sr_10/sr10_257.pdf.

CHAPTER 1

1   Phillippa Lally et al., "How Are Habits Formed: Modelling Habit Formation in the Real World," *European Journal of Social Psychology* 40 (2010): 998–1009. Published online 16 July 2009 in Wiley Online Library. http://repositorio.ispa.pt/bitstream/10400.12/3364/1/IJSP_998-1009.pdf

2   Gregory D. Lewis et al., "Metabolic Signatures of Exercise in Human Plasma," *Science Translational Medicine* 2 (May 26, 2010): 33–37. http://stm.sciencemag.org/content/2/33/33ra37

3   M. Ayabe et al., "Very Short Bouts of Non-Exercise Daily Physical Activity Is Associated with Lower Visceral Fat in Japanese Female Adults," *European Journal of Applied Physiology* 112 (2012): 3525. http://link.springer.com/article/10.1007/s00421-012-2342-8

4   Jenna B. Gillen et al., "Three Minutes of All-Out Intermittent Exercise per Week Increases Skeletal Muscle Oxidative Capacity and Improves Cardiometabolic Health," *PLoS One* 9 (November 2014): e111489. http://www.ncbi.nlm.nih.gov/pmc/articles/PMC4218754/

5   T. S. Church, C. P. Earnest, J. S. Skinner, and S. N. Blair, "Effects of Different Doses of Physical Activity on Cardiorespiratory Fitness among Sedentary, Overweight, or Obese Postmenopausal Women with Elevated Blood Pressure: A Randomized Controlled Trial," *JAMA* 297, no. 1 (May 16, 2007): 2081–91.

6   A. B. Sullivan, E. Covington, and J. Scheman, "Immediate Benefits of a Brief 10-Minute Exercise Protocol in a Chronic Pain Population: A Pilot Study," *Pain Med* 11 (2010): 524–29. http://painmedicine.oxfordjournals.org/content/11/4/524.long

7   Attila Szabo, Zoltan Gaspar, and Julia Abraham, "Acute Effects of Light Exercise on Subjectively Experienced Well-Being: Benefits in Only Three Minutes," *Baltic Journal of Health & Physical Activity* 5 (December 2013): 261. https://www.researchgate.net/publication/260293190_Acute_effects_of_light_exercise_on_subjectively_experienced_well-being_Benefits_in_only_three_minutes

8   L. L. Andersen et al., "Effect of Brief Daily Exercise on Headaches among Adults—Secondary Analysis of a Randomized Controlled Trial," *Scandinavian Journal of Work, Environment, & Health* 37 (November 2011): 547–50. http://www.ncbi.nlm.nih.gov/pubmed/21617837

9   Deanne McArthur et al., "Factors Influencing Adherence to Regular Exercise in Middle-Aged Women: A Qualitative Study to Inform Clinical Practice," *BMC Women's Health* 14 (2014): 49. http://www.ncbi.nlm.nih.gov/pmc/articles/PMC3975263/

10 C. Jeng, S. H. Yang, P. C. Chang, and L. I. Tsao, "Menopausal Women: Perceiving Continuous Power through the Experience of Regular Exercise," *Journal of Clinical Nursing* 13 (May 2004): 447–54. http://www.ncbi.nlm.nih.gov/pubmed/15086631

11 A. Golay et al., "Taking Small Steps towards Targets—Perspectives for Clinical Practice in Diabetes, Cardiometabolic Disorders and Beyond," *International Journal of Clinical Practice* 67 (April 1, 2013): 322–32. https://www.ncbi.nlm.nih.gov/pubmed/23521324

CHAPTER 2

1   T. Mann, A. J. Tomiyama, E. Westling, et al., "Medicare's Search for Effective Obesity Treatments: Diets Are Not the Answer," *American Psychologist* 62, no. 3 (April 2007): 220–33.

2   Jean Fain, "In 'Eating Lab,' a Psychologist Spills Secrets on Why Diets Fail," NPR, June 1, 2015. http://www.npr.org/sections/thesalt/2015/06/01/411217634/in-eating-lab-psychologist-spills-secrets-on-why-diets-fail

3   Jack F. Hollis et al., "Weight Loss During the Intensive Intervention Phase of the Weight-Loss Maintenance Trial," *American Journal of Preventive Medicine* 35 (August 2008): 118–26. http://www.ncbi.nlm.nih.gov/pmc/articles/PMC2515566/

CHAPTER 3

1   J. G. LaRose et al., "Differences in Motivations and Weight Loss Behaviors in Young Adults and Older Adults in the National Weight Control Registry," *Obesity* 21 (2013): 449–53. https://www.ncbi.nlm.nih.gov/pmc/articles/PMC3630273/

2 A. A. Gorin et al., "Medical Triggers Are Associated with Better Short- and Long-Term Weight Loss Outcomes," *Preventive Medicine* 39 (2004): 612–16. https://www.ncbi.nlm.nih.gov/pubmed/15313102

3 L. R. Vartanian, K. Kernan, and B. Wansink, "Clutter, Chaos, and Overconsumption: The Role of Mind-Set in Stressful and Chaotic Food Environments," *Environment and Behavior* (2016). http://eab.sagepub.com/content/early/2016/01/28/0013916516628178.abstract

4 J. E. Painter et al., "How Visibility and Convenience Influence Candy Consumption," *Appetite* 38 (June 2002): 237–38. (cited in Vartanian, "Clutter, Chaos, and Overconsumption")

5 C. J. Metzgar et al., "Facilitators and Barriers to Weight Loss and Weight Loss Maintenance: A Qualitative Exploration," *Journal of Human Nutrition and Dietetics* 28 (2015): 593–603. http://www.readcube.com/articles/10.1111/jhn.12273

6 M. L. Wang, L. Pbert, and S. C. Lemon, "Influence of Family, Friend and Coworker Social Support and Social Undermining on Weight Gain Prevention among Adults," *Obesity* 22 (2014): 1973–80. http://onlinelibrary.wiley.com/doi/10.1002/oby.20814/full

7 Ibid.

8 Dori M. Steinberg, Gary G. Bennett, Sandy Askew, and Deborah F. Tate, "Weighing Every Day Matters: Daily Weighing Improves Weight Loss and Adoption of Weight Control Behaviors," *Journal of the Academy of Nutrition and Dietetics* 115, no. 4 (April 2015): 511–18.

9 C. R. Pacanowski, F. C. Bertz, and D. A. Levitsky, "Daily Self-Weighing to Control Body Weight in Adults: A Critical Review of the Literature," *Sage Open* 4, no. 4 (October-December 2014): 1–16.

10 Karen L. Smith-Janssen, "Should You Weigh Yourself Every Day?" *Prevention* (June 22, 2015). http://www.prevention.com/weight-loss/daily-weigh-ins

11 Metzgar et al., 593–603.

12 E. B. Loucks, W. B. Britton, C. J. Howe, et al., "Associations of Dispositional Mindfulness with Obesity and Central Adiposity: The New England Family Study," *International Journal of Behavioral Medicine* 23, no. 2 (April 2016): 224–33.

13 Colby Itkowitz, "Mind over Meal: Study Reveals a Weight Loss Strategy You May Never Have Considered," *Washington Post* (October 22, 2015). https://www.washingtonpost.com/news/inspired-life/wp/2015/10/22/could-practicing-mindfulness-reduce-belly-fat/

14 Metzgar et al., 593–603.

CHAPTER 4

1 B. S. Shaw et al., "Anthropometric and Cardiovascular Responses to Hypertrophic Resistance Training in Postmenopausal Women," *Menopause* (July 18, 2016). http://www.ncbi.nlm.nih.gov/pubmed/27433861

2 K. R. Baker et al., "The Efficacy of Home-Based Progressive Strength Training in Older Adults with Knee Osteoarthritis: A Randomized Controlled Trial," *Journal of Rheumatology* 28 (2001): 1655–65. https://www.ncbi.nlm.nih.gov/pubmed/11469475

3 Robert T. Kell and Gordon J. Asmundson, "A Comparison of Two Forms of Periodized Exercise Rehabilitation Programs in the Management of Chronic Nonspecific Low-Back Pain," *Journal of Strength & Conditioning Research* 23 (March 2009): 513–23. http://journals.lww.com/nsca-jscr/pages/articleviewer.aspx?year=2009&issue=03000&article=00022&type=abstract

4 Ginny Graves, "Your Muscles, Your Life," *Prevention* (November 2014).

5 Teresa Liu-Ambrose, "Reversing Cognitive Decline through Resistance Training," University of British Columbia (April 23, 2012). http://www.med.ubc.ca/reversing-cognitive-decline-through-resistance-training/

6 H. Kaikkonen et al., "The Effect of Heart Rate Controlled Low Resistance Circuit Weight Training and Endurance Training on Maximal Aerobic Power in Sedentary Adults," *Scandinavian Journal of Medicine & Science in Sports* 10 (2000): 211–15. https://www.ncbi.nlm.nih.gov/pubmed/10898265

7 Nina J. Kise et al., "Exercise Therapy versus Arthroscopic Partial Meniscectomy for Degenerative Meniscal Tear in Middle Aged Patients: Randomised Controlled Trial with Two Year Follow-Up," *BMJ* 354 (July 20, 2016): i3740.

8 K. Bailey and M. Jung, "The Early Bird Gets the Worm! Congruency Between Intentions and Behavior Is Highest When Plans to Exercise Are Made for the Morning," *Journal of Applied Biobehavioral Research* 19 (December 3, 2014): 233–47. http://onlinelibrary.wiley.com/doi/10.1111/jabr.12027/abstract

9 Karen J. Sherman et al., "A Randomized Trial Comparing Yoga, Stretching, and a Self-Care Book for Chronic Low Back Pain," *Archives of Internal Medicine* 171 (December 12, 2011): 2019–26. http://www.ncbi.nlm.nih.gov/pmc/articles/PMC3279296/

CHAPTER 6

1 "Sugar 101," American Heart Association (August 29, 2016). www.heart.org/HEARTORG/HealthyLiving/HealthyEating/Nutrition/Sugar-101_UCM_306024_Article.jsp#.V3L0dOYrJsM

2 "Carbohydrates and Blood Sugar," Harvard T. H. Chan School of Public Health (June 28, 2016). https://www.hsph.harvard.edu/nutritionsource/carbohydrates/carbohydrates-and-blood-sugar/

3 P. M. Wise et al., "Reduced Dietary Intake of Simple Sugars Alters Perceived Sweet Taste Intensity But Not Perceived Pleasantness," *American Journal of Clinical Nutrition* 103 (January 2016): 50–60. http://www.ncbi.nlm.nih.gov/pubmed/26607941

4 "Can Eating Fruits and Vegetables Help People to Manage Their Weight?" *National Center for Chronic Disease Prevention and Health Promotion* (July 2, 2016). http://www.cdc.gov/nccdphp/dnpa/nutrition/pdf/rtp_practitioner_10_07.pdf

5 Markham Heid, "What You Should Really Be Looking for on a Nutrition Label," *Prevention* (December 22, 2014). http://www.prevention.com/food/healthy-eating-tips/how-read-food-labels

6 "Changes to the Nutrition Facts Label," US Food and Drug Administration (December 22, 2014). http://www.fda.gov/Food/GuidanceRegulation/GuidanceDocumentsRegulatoryInformation/LabelingNutrition/ucm385663.htm#images

7 B. Batemen et al., "The Effects of a Double Blind, Placebo Controlled, Artificial Food Colourings, and Benzoate Preservative Challenge on Hyperactivity in a General Population Sample of Preschool Children," *Archives of Disease in Childhood* 89 (2004): 506–11. http://adc.bmj.com/content/89/6/506.short

8 The United States Healthful Food Council Web site: http://ushfc.org/about/#fancy-form-delay

9 "Estimated Calorie Needs per Day by Age, Gender, and Physical Activity Level," http://www.cnpp.usda.gov/sites/default/files/usda_food_patterns/EstimatedCalorieNeedsPerDayTable.pdf

10 V. E. Fernandez-Elias et al., "Ingestion of a Moderately High Caffeine Dose before Exercise Increases Postexercise Energy Expenditure," *International Journal of Sport, Nutrition, and Exercise Metabolism* 25 (February 2015): 46–53. http://www.ncbi.nlm.nih.gov/pubmed/24901809

11 International Delight Web site: https://www.internationaldelight.com/products/french-vanilla

12 L. D. Whigham, A. C. Watras, and D. A. Schoeller, "Efficacy of Conjugated Linoleic Acid for Reducing Fat Mass: A Meta-Analysis in Humans," *American Journal of Clinical Nutrition* 85 (May 2007): 1203–11. http://www.ncbi.nlm.nih.gov/pubmed/17490954

13 Dominika Srednicka-Tober et al., "Higher PUFA and n-3 PUFA, Conjugated Linoleic Acid, α-Tocopherol and Iron, but Lower Iodine and Selenium Concentrations in Organic Milk: A Systematic Literature Review and Meta- and Redundancy Analyses," *British Journal of Nutrition* 115 (March 2016): 1043–60. http://journals.cambridge.org/download.php?file=%2FBJN%2FBJN115_06%2FS0007114516000349a.pdf&code=d5a1b665aceb8052f111c69b82140018

14 30 x 2 servings (who uses just 1 tablespoon?)= 60; 60 x 2 cups = 120 calories; 120 cals x 365 days = 43,800; 43,800 divided by 3,500 = 12.5ish

15 The Environmental Working Group, "Executive Summary: EWG's 2016 Shopper's Guide to Pesticides in Produce" (June 28, 2016). https://www.ewg.org/foodnews/summary.php

16 The Environmental Working Group, "Clean Fifteen" (June 28, 2016). https://www.ewg.org/foodnews/clean_fifteen_list.php

17 The Environmental Working Group, "Dirty Dozen" (June 28, 2016). https://www.ewg.org/foodnews/dirty_dozen_list.php

18 J. Suez et al., "Artificial Sweeteners Induce Glucose Intolerance by Altering the Gut Microbiota," *Nature* (published online September 17, 2014). http://www.nature.com/nature/journal/vaop/ncurrent/full/nature13793.html

19 Stephanie Ecklecamp, "Is Gelatin the Next Big Superfood?" *Prevention* (March 12, 2015). http://www.prevention.com/food/gelatin-superfood

20 K. Jaceldo-Siegl et al., "Tree Nuts Are Inversely Associated with Metabolic Syndrome and Obesity: The Adventist Health Study," *PLOS ONE* (January 8, 2014). http://journals.plos.org/plosone/article?id=10.1371/journal.pone.0085133

21 T. A. Churchward-Venne et al., "Nutritional Regulation of Muscle Protein Synthesis with Resistance Exercise: Strategies to Enhance Anabolism," *Nutrition & Metabolism* 10 (May 17, 2012). http://www.ncbi.nlm.nih.gov/pmc/articles/PMC3464665/

22 M. Iizuka et al., "Inhibitory Effects of Balsamic Vinegar on LDL Oxidation and Lipid Accumulation in THP-1 Macrophages," *Journal of Nutritional Science & Vitaminology* 56 (2010): 421–27. http://www.ncbi.nlm.nih.gov/pubmed/21422711

23 R. Vidavalur et al., "Significance of Wine and Resveratrol in Cardiovascular Disease: French Paradox Revisited," *Experimental Cardiology* 11 (Fall 2006): 217–25. http://www.ncbi.nlm.nih.gov/pmc/articles/PMC2276147/

24 "What You Need to Know About Mercury in Fish and Shellfish," FDA brochure (June 28, 2016). http://www.fda.gov/food/resourcesforyou/consumers/ucm110591.htm

25 Jean L. Kristeller and Ruth Q. Wolever, "Mindfulness-Based Eating Awareness Training for Treating Binge-Eating Disorder: The Conceptual Foundation," *Eating Disorders* 19 (December 20, 2010): 49–61. http://www.indstate.edu/cas/sites/arts.indstate.edu/files/Psychology/Kristeller_Wolever_ED_Conceptual_Paper.pdf

CHAPTER 7

1 W. Westcott et al., "Nutrition Programs Enhance Exercise Effects on Body Composition and Resting Blood Pressure," *The Physician and Sports Medicine* 41 (September 2013). https://www.acefitness.org/continuingeducation/courses/support_items/OLC-PSM-NPEEE/NutritionJuly2014.pdf

2 Michael Boschmann et al., "Water-Induced Thermogenesis," *Journal of Clinical Endocrinology and Metabolism* 88, no. 12 (December 2003): 6015–9.

3 G. Dubnov-Raz et al., "Influence of Water Drinking on Resting Energy Expenditure in Overweight Children," *International Journal of Obesity* 35 (October 2011): 1295–1300.

Index

Underscored page references indicate boxed text.
Boldface page references indicate photographs.
An asterisk (*) indicates recipe photos are shown in the color insert.